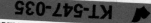
Nursing, medicine and primary care

Open University Press
Buckingham • Philadelphia

Open University Press
Celtic Court
22 Ballmoor
Buckingham
MK18 1XW

email: enquiries@openup.co.uk
world wide web: www.openup.co.uk

and

325 Chestnut Street
Philadelphia, PA 19106, USA

First Published 2000

A catalogue record of this book is available from the British Library

ISBN   0 335 20167 9 (pb)   0 335 20168 7 (hb)

Library of Congress Cataloging-in-Publication Data
Williams, Anne, 1994–
    Nursing, medicine, and primary care / Anne Williams.
       p. cm.
    Includes bibliographical references and index.
    ISBN 0-335-20168-7 (hb) – ISBN 0-335-20167-9 (pbk.)
    1. Nurse and physician–Great Britain.   2. Primary care (Medicine)–Great Britain.   I. Title.
  RT86.4.W54 2000
  362.1'0941–dc21   99-049874

Typeset by Graphicraft Limited, Hong Kong
Printed in Great Britain by Biddles Ltd, Guildford and King's Lynn

For my parents, Bill and Linda Williams

Contents

Acknowledgements

I wish to acknowledge the National Primary Care Research and Development Centre, University of Manchester for its financial support of the research project, 'Cultural differences between medicine and nursing and implications for primary care'. I should also record my thanks to colleagues in the School of Nursing, Midwifery and Health Visiting, University of Manchester, who kindly allowed me to devote time to the project. Bonnie Sibbald has provided constant support throughout, and I am especially grateful to her for the chapter she has contributed to this book. Thanks are also due to Mary Black, Caroline Glendinning, Jackie Hayden, Sue Kirk, Carl May, Tamasine Robins, Anne Rogers, Martin Roland, Steve Rose and David Wilkin. I would like to pay special tribute to those who agreed to participate in the research and who gave so freely of their experience and knowledge of primary care.

Since my appointment to the School of Health Science, University of Wales Swansea, I have received further encouragement. I am indebted to Barbara Green, Director of the School, for her generous support and to other colleagues within the School for their insightful comments on drafts of chapters and for the many helpful conversations. Thanks to you all, including June Clark, David Hughes, David Greaves, Martyn Evans and, especially, Sue Sullivan for her insights into patients' perspectives. Her sharp sociological eye has been invaluable and her courage an inspiration. I have also benefited from discussions with staff, practitioners and research students within the 'Changing roles and relations in health care' research group, notably Alison Hughes, Melanie Jones, Joy Merrell, Sarah Osborne, Sue Philpin, Anne Price, Denise Rogers, Julie Slater, Paul Wainwright and Tessa Watts.

A key moment in the evolution of the book was the response of the anonymous reviewers to the research report and proposed book. Their full and helpful criticisms gave me the confidence to proceed. Many thanks to all four reviewers. Thanks also to Blackwell Science for permission to reproduce data from pages 737–45 from volume 29:3 of *Journal of Advanced Nursing*.

Over the years, a number of people have influenced my understanding of the issues and myriad ideas which inform the book's argument. Some are acknowledged, in conventional manner, in the text and references. Even so, there remain others whose work is not immediately and obviously critical to the discussion within these covers but to whom, nevertheless, I owe a considerable debt of gratitude. I would particularly like to record thanks to the following: David Morgan, Department of Sociology, University of Manchester; Liz Stanley, Women's Studies, University of Manchester; and Elvi Whittaker, Department of Anthropology and Sociology, University of British Columbia, Canada.

Finally, thanks to my parents for their unfailing encouragement and inspiration over many years and to my husband, Bernard Curtis, for his scholarly advice, material support and for bearing the brunt of my preoccupation with the book with such good grace.

Anne Williams
School of Health Science
University of Wales Swansea

Introduction

This is a book about cultural differences between medicine and nursing and implications for primary care. It takes as its starting point the view that doctors and nurses have strong passions about their various contributions to the health of society, and it is concerned with how professional ideas and interests are to be weighed against the need to operate a system that works for the greater good of society. The book draws substantially on empirical work including a literature review undertaken to explore this dimension of health care provision (Williams *et al.* 1997). This introduction sets the scene for discussion, identifies relevant concepts, introduces the major themes of the chapters that follow and comments on the methodology of the empirical work.

Changing health care scenes

Health work has been at the cutting edge of a politically inspired attempt to restructure working practices in Britain over the last decade. Attempts at creating markets, giving priority to consumers over producers, introducing new forms of management and cost containment, have turned the health service into a laboratory of experimentation in changing work practices.

(Walby *et al.* 1994)

These words were written in the wake of organizational changes to the health service set out in the White Paper *Working for Patients* (Department of Health 1989) and made law through the NHS and Community Care Act 1990. Changes stemmed from the 1979–97 Conservative government's programme of economic and institutional reforms, based on the idea of a free market economy. The reforms encompassed new management structures, including flexible employment, new forms of financial control and strategic planning (Keat and Abercrombie 1991). The implementation of the reforms 'fundamentally altered the structuring and functioning of the NHS' (Flynn *et al.* 1996) and as Walby and her colleagues (1994) suggest, the transition from one set of working practices to another was hardly smooth. New issues arising from the changes were colliding with old lines of conflict in the health professions. Increasing emphasis on the relationship between producers and consumers crossed paths with traditional conflicts between bureaucrats and professionals, not least at the intersection between medicine and nursing.

Since publication in 1994 of *Medicine and Nursing: Professions in a Changing Health Service*, the changing health care scene observed by Walby and her colleagues has intensified at the point of intersection between the professions of medicine and nursing. Anxious to promote a successful internal market in health care provision and to contain costs, the 1979–97 Conservative government continued to apply pressure to improve the cost-effectiveness of health delivery, focusing attention on the possible benefits of moving some areas of health care work and responsibility from expensive to cheaper health care providers, in particular from doctors to nurses (Richardson and Maynard 1995). Key factors in this process were the introduction of the reduction of junior hospital doctors' hours, falls in the general practitioner (GP) workforce – a result of declining recruitment to the speciality – increased retirement rates and a move towards part-time working favoured by the increasing proportion of women in medicine (Carlisle and Johnstone 1996, Taylor and Leese 1997). Since the change of government in 1997, Labour has continued to drive a programme of reform departing in some critical respects from the reforms set in train by the Conservative government. There is greater emphasis on ideas about collaboration and partnership rather than on competition (Department of Health 1998; Welsh Office 1998a), and on 'patients' as opposed to 'consumers of care' – a policy drive and associated rhetoric that mark a major shift in thinking about the organization of care. Nonetheless, as argued throughout this book, the competitive legacy of the free market reforms remains, and consumerism is still highly influential. As with the Conservatives, Labour's agenda embodies a managed health service – an agenda which does not sit easily with ideas about professional autonomy and interests.

It is against this backdrop of rapidly changing scenes and competing ideas that this book seeks to elucidate cultural differences between medicine and nursing, and implications for primary care. The following chapters focus on changing boundaries and relationships between the two professions, exploring ways in which ideas and values are used to establish, maintain and justify professional identities. In this respect it is a book about similarities and differences between, as well as diversity across and within, the two professions.

There are a number of analyses which deal with boundary issues and relationships between medicine and nursing. Those contained within the

covers of sociological texts have a theoretical edge which assists an understanding of the differences between the two professions, many highlighting
how social context, power, and the variables of class, gender and race structure relationships (see, for example, Witz 1992; Mackay 1993; Walby *et al.*
1994; Davies 1995; Porter 1995; Wicks 1998). However, interest in relationships between the two professions is not confined to theoretical accounts, as
the soap operas and documentaries on our television screens demonstrate.
The latter present colourful constructions of everyday life in the field of
health care inspired by 'real' doctors and nurses engaged in the collective
struggle to give meaning and purpose to life events such as birth, illness and
death. Common to both sociological and media accounts is a preference for
the acute and the urgent in health care. Sociological accounts have dealt
almost exclusively with boundaries and relationships between the two
professions in the context of the hospital. Notable examples include Walby
et al. (1994) in the British context, and, very recently, Wicks (1998) in the
Australian context. The same is true for television soap operas, perhaps most
obviously *Casualty* and *ER*. Certainly, the hospital is a focus of abiding interest where lives are lost – or saved, often through dramatic interventions.

Spotlight on primary care

In some contrast, this book features what might at first glance appear to be
a pallid setting, that of the British primary care system – the point of first
contact with a health practitioner. It is a setting where health is promoted,
chronic conditions are managed and serious acute illness is normally referred to medical consultants who are located predominantly in hospitals.
Primary care is a setting which to date has received little attention in the
literature dealing with interoccupational matters, although authors such as
Flynn *et al.* (1996) have addressed issues such as the organization of the
relationship between primary care and community health services. Ironic-
ally, however, it is the relatively humdrum setting of primary care that has
been chosen to lead the National Health Service (NHS) into the future.

   With the spotlight on primary care, we can see that at its heart lie issues
of political significance to policy makers, professionals and workforce managers concerning who leads and who follows in the new emerging health
service. As noted in the following chapters, there is a degree of insecurity
about this, fostered in some respects by the increasing movement of areas of
work and responsibility from doctors to nurses. Perhaps more importantly,
insecurity has been fostered by the vigorous efforts of general management
to exercise more control over the health care workforce. These processes
have heightened professional sensitivities so that primary care, in the UK at
least, has become the scene of potential drama at all levels, where ideas
about partnership and collaboration (Department of Health 1998; Welsh
Office 1998a, b, c) confront the competitive legacy of the market, and where

enterprise and self-interest (Keat and Abercrombie 1991) jostle with ideas about meeting need and empowering patients.

Some might even argue that there is an element of tragedy as they survey the changing primary care scene. For while general practice medicine may feel confident in facing the future given the policy commitment to a primary-care-led National Health Service, some individual general practitioners have experienced a sense of loss as work moves from doctors to nurses. The situation is even more ambiguous for nurses. On the one hand, there is a sense of excitement around changes in policy makers' expectations of nurses and subsequent future possibilities; on the other, nurses continue to be affected by their subordinate position as a profession, in relation to medicine. While nurses will have the opportunity to participate in the new decision-making groups, for example local health groups (LHGs) in Wales and primary health groups (PHGs) in England, and their equivalents else-where, they are unlikely to take the overall lead in at least the immediate future, and their numbers in these critical groups are fewer than those of general practitioners. Added to which, nursing confidence continues to be eroded by uncertainties in respect of nurse education.

Commenting on educational reforms in the 1980s, Davies (1995: 113) posed the question, 'Did anyone outside nursing really want a better educated nurse?' She went on to suggest that 'there were some at least in the medical profession who were prepared to say outright that they did not', and provides convincing evidence to support her comment (pp. 113–16), prefacing her discussion with the proviso that negative medical commentary at the time was in no way representative of the views of the medical profession as a whole or indeed any section of it. In the various explorations which underpin discussion within this book, commentary by individual doctors has been unanimously supportive of improved provision for nurse education. However, in the wake of the recent educational gains for nursing, not least the move of nursing into higher education, nurses continue to encounter ostensibly ad hoc opposition to their new-found gains, as discussed in later chapters.

UK primary care

It is important to emphasize that the setting for the book's discussion is the UK primary care system, conceived as first point of contact for health care for most of the population. As discussed by Roland and Wilkin (1996: 7) health care is provided by 'generalists rather than specialists with a broad range of competencies suited to dealing with both well defined and undifferentiated problems'. Important amongst the particular features of care provided by generalists, as Roland and Wilkin suggest, is that care emphasizes the whole person and the context in which that person lives, it is person centred as opposed to disease centred, provides continuity of care over a long period of time and coordinates care for individual patients. Primary care in respect of these features encompasses ideas and values shared by both nurses and doctors internationally.

As noted throughout the book but especially in Chapter 3, there are significant differences between the professions in relation to the ways in which ideas and values are interpreted, as indeed there are differences within professional groups. Similarly, the political context within which primary care is practised makes a difference. The emphasis in UK primary care, as implied by Roland and Wilkin, is on persons. In this respect its focus is narrower than that of World Health Organization primary 'health care' which encompasses a concern with populations as well as individuals (World Health Organization 1978, 1991). Arguably, the recent drive to integrate elements of the public health agenda into primary care (for example, Primary Care Network 1998) as well as the incorporation of 'community approaches to primary care' (for example, Health Promotion Wales 1998) will make a difference to the UK emphasis. As we shall see, especially in Chapter 5, some nurses tend to appeal to ideas about public health and community approaches in order to distinguish their contribution to primary care from that of general practitioners.

The main players

As will be evident from the preceding discussion, the main players in the present discussion of cultural differences between medicine and nursing are doctors and nurses working in primary care within the UK. Doctors constitute a professional group which is far from monolithic. General practitioners differ from physicians and surgeons in their history and ethos, a point discussed in detail in Chapter 1. Nurses, however, take centre stage, mainly insofar as at the outset of the study which informs the discussion contained within this book (Williams *et al.* 1997), there was a real concern that policies which encourage nurses to undertake work formerly performed by doctors might erode nursing autonomy and undermine its sense of professional identity, so impoverishing the quality of patient care. However, it was thought also plausible that such new dimensions to role and work might enable nurses to achieve greater autonomy and an ability to bring their values to bear on a wider range of health services (Sibbald 1996: 33). While a number of studies demonstrated that work was moving from doctors to nurses and explored the policy drivers and economic ramifications, few studies had reflected on how ideas, values and beliefs were being challenged. It was considered timely to attempt such an analysis. The study was undertaken at the National Primary Care Research and Development Centre (NPCRDC), University of Manchester, and is referred to as the NPCRDC study in the remainder of the book.

Nurses do not constitute a homogeneous group, and there is considerable role variation between primary care nurses. Role is a slippery concept, signifying function – a job of work, a part to play – upon which are consequent a number of relationships. Practice nurses and those nurses working in primary care and designated 'nurse practitioners' (Royal College of Nursing 1997) may share many interests; even so, each group is viewed as different from the other in respect of role. For while both may be expanding their roles, practice nurses have traditionally been associated with delegated work supervised by general practitioners, while nurse practitioners have been associated with role substitution where work and responsibilities pass from doctor to nurse. At all events, there is a degree of ambiguity around ideas about delegation and nurse/doctor substitution, as discussed in Chapter 2 and elsewhere in the book.

There are also distinctions to be made between, on the one hand, nurses strongly affiliated to general practice such as practice nurses and nurse practitioners and, on the other, community nurses – health visitors and district nurses. The latter, both with origins in the north west of England, share a history of working with patients and clients in their homes as well as in health centres and practices (Robertson 1991). Nevertheless, there are significant differences between district nurses and health visitors. The former work mainly with an ill population whereas the latter work with a well population and are strongly influenced by the idea of public health. District nurses have tended to be subject to direction from general practitioners whereas health visitors have had their own case loads. It is also possible for a community nurse to be a nurse practitioner: for example, a health visitor may also work as a nurse practitioner having obtained the appropriate training and education at either undergraduate or postgraduate degree level. As observed in Chapter 3 there are contractual differences in respect of all categories of nurses which affect their relationships with each other and with general practitioners, especially when new roles are created.

As for other players in primary care – patients, carers, policy makers, managers, educationists, other professionals and workers – most are assigned to no more than a walk-on part in the following chapters, although nurses and doctors interviewed for the NPCRDC study included nurses who managed other nurses, taught nurses and made policy. Similarly, the doctors interviewed included those who organized general practitioner training. We did not interview members of other professional groups in health and social care. Patients' comments on cultural differences between medicine and nursing were sought. The literature search included seeking out patients' views and a commentator was interviewed about consumer views. The designation 'consumer' rather than 'patient', 'client' or 'member of the public' reflects the ethos of health services research in 1996, the point when the study commenced. More recently, the word 'patient' appears to be gaining currency outside the hospital. There are policy drives to give greater priority to patients' views on health matters (for example, Welsh Office 1998a, b) and patient involvement in clinical decision making is seen as a distinct possibility, though not without problems (Sullivan and Pickering 1997). 'The patient' makes a brief appearance in this book, and there is a sense in which patient perspectives on cultural differences between medicine and nursing and implications for primary care are barely rehearsed, though recent policy drives to 'increasing the role of individuals, patients and carers in their health care ... and encourage lay perspectives to inform research' may make a difference (Welsh Office 1998b, c, d).

Shared scripts? Culture, difference and inequality

Ideas and values are the currency of culture. As noted above, and discussed in some detail throughout the book, in common with the rest of society nurses and doctors working in primary care share culture. For example, general practitioners as well as nurses identify with the idea of the whole person and taking a holistic perspective. In Chapter 3 the differences in orientation and interpretation of holism are considered – and there are significant differences in this respect between nurses and doctors, as we shall see. All the same, the idea of holism is recognized and shared, as are ideas about curing as well as care, compassion and concern for the common good. Similarly, ideas associated with enterprise culture including the consumerism and competition of 'commercial enterprise' and the enterprising qualities of initiative, energy and independence (Keat 1991: 3) are available to both medicine and nursing.

What is also shared is the organization of ideas. LeVine, an anthropologist writing in 1986, suggests that the shared organization of ideas includes the intellectual, moral and aesthetic standards prevalent in a community and the meanings of communicative actions (LeVine 1986: 66–77). Thus, he says, it is important for those investigating culture to take account of general rules, concepts or assumptions that generate the particulars readily accessible to the investigator. The concept of community can be understood in a number of sometimes overlapping ways. These include community defined as a geographical area and community defined as a network of interests. LeVine discovered a supra-individual, collective script when exploring how intense emotional experiences were reported in the geographical community he was studying in Kenya between 1946 and 1949. To take examples closer to the current discussion, an exploration of the particulars of the history of ideas constituting western medicine suggests that ideas about health and illness are organized around a taken-for-granted separation between mind and body. Thus distinctions are drawn between, for example, psychiatry and medicine. Correspondingly, distinctions are drawn between 'psychiatric or mental health nursing' and 'nursing'. The mind/body dichotomy may be contested, it may be displaced, but only insofar as another conceptualization shared and recognized by a community is strong enough to dislodge it. As already suggested, conceptions of primary care constitute another area of debate. The important point is that it is the shared ideas, values, hopes and aspirations informing debate which give a community or group character and identity. From this perspective, while there may be differences of standpoint, it is possible to argue that there are no fundamental cultural differences between nurses and doctors. Rather, nurses and doctors are viewed as part of a common community of health care, each profession subject to similar contraints imposed by the economics and politics of the age.

The problem with this perspective is that it does not take into account the dynamics of culture. Difference lies partly in how values and ideas are interpreted and used by individuals who in turn are influenced by their historical and contemporary circumstances. And as Lupton (1995) observes, the circumstances of our society include an economic and political system which relies on personal, moral responsibility for individual prosperity and self-actualization. The emphasis on personal responsibility is the legacy of individualism, a prominent feature of Enlightenment thinking and one which has remained highly influential ever since. Individualism has been used to justify policies which aim to improve states of being – such as the state of 'being healthy' (for example, the 'Look after yourself' campaign of the mid-1980s). It has also been used to justify policies which aim to change behaviour in order to improve, for example, the 'efficiency' and 'effectiveness' of organizations, bearing in mind that these concepts are contested on the grounds that there is more than one way of construing what counts as efficiency and effectiveness (Holland 1983; Øvretveit 1998; St Leger *et al.* 1992), a point noted in Chapter 2 and again in Chapter 5 in relation to the cost-effectiveness of new and changing roles in primary care nursing.

Readers will be aware of the sociological critique of individualism, which is to emphasize the mediating effects of environmental or structural variables such as class, age, location, race and sex in shaping the experiences of people – including the differential experiences of nurses and doctors. The critique also takes into account the dynamics of identity – the construction of boundaries between us and them, self and other, general practitioner and hospital doctor, doctor and nurse, primary care nurse and community nurse and so on. Power is the critical factor at play in the processes of interplay between, on the one hand, action and agency and, on the other, the factors structural and otherwise which constrain. From this perspective, the fundamental difference between medicine and nursing is the difference in professional status and power. Earlier in the discussion it was noted how individual doctors may feel a sense of loss and insecurity about areas of work and responsibility moving to nursing, a point explored in later chapters. Yet, medicine as a profession continues to enjoy power and influence. In contrast, while individual nurses may feel a sense of excitement about new possibilities, the enduring insecurity for the nursing profession has been intimately tied to lack of power, specifically in relation to its subordinate position in relation to medicine.

In the chapters which follow, power is a key factor in discussions pertaining to cultural differences. Chapter 1 'Background and policy issues' focuses at the outset on the play for power at the boundary between hospital medicine and general practice. It is observed that the cultural identity of general practice medicine has been largely forged in relation to hospital medicine and with appeal to the defining notion of generalist, as opposed to specialist, practice. Discussion then turns to the successive policy and contractual changes governing the development of general practice medicine and more generally primary care. It is argued that while the substitution of doctors by nurses challenges the generalist role of the primary care physician, policy changes have favoured medicine rather than nursing. In Chapter 2 'Boundary changes in primary care' the spotlight falls on the boundary between medicine and nursing in order to illuminate boundary changes between the two professions. The notion of role substitution is viewed from a variety of perspectives, and the play for power between professional groups is noted. Elements of the wider context in which this play for power occurs are discussed, not least the efforts of general management to constrain processes of professionalization. In Chapter 3 'Working on the boundaries' the complexities of how boundaries are constructed and professional identities maintained are elucidated. Reference is made to values and ideas held in common by the two professions and how they are interpreted and treated differently, a process which contributes to their distinguishing features. The chapter concludes by identifying a set of ideas loosely associated with professional identity and purpose which is set against ideas linked with 'enterprise culture'. The juxtaposition of the two sets of ideas, it is suggested, makes for a situation of vulnerability and uncertainty, especially for primary care nurses. This situation is explored in some detail in Chapter 4 'Boundary culture: exploring a realm of uncertainty'. It is suggested that nursing leaders and other health policy makers must acknowledge factors that undermine a clear, confident nursing contribution to primary care, not least the erosion of a sense of professional identity.

Paradoxical as it may seem, uncertainty has the potential to inspire innovation as well as to undermine it. This point is taken up in Chapter 5 where it is argued that innovation rests, in part at least, in striking a balance between enterprise together with its associated values and the need for a clear sense of professional identity. The implications of this argument for innovation in primary care are discussed in detail. Key points of discussion include the preconditions for innovation, the need to foster interprofessional collaboration and the likelihood of better outcomes for patients. In the final chapter the point is made that differences between the two professions, especially the difference in status, will have implications for taking forward a primary care agenda where the emphasis is on cooperation, partnership and collaboration. This is because effective cooperation depends on a nursing workforce which has confidence in its contribution to primary care. A discussion of how such confidence might be encouraged brings the book to a conclusion.

The research study in outline

Discussion in this book stems from a concern to better understand the contribution of nursing to the changing primary care scene. It owes much to the NPCRDC study undertaken in order to identify core values in nursing and to consider how such values differ from those of medicine (Williams *et al.* 1997). The study aimed to explore what distinctive aspects of care may be lost or gained as primary care nurses take on work formerly the province of general practitioners. From the outset of the study, an understanding of these areas of concern was considered essential to inform policy development, to guide the management of skill mix change, and to plan evaluations of the cost-effectiveness of nurse/doctor substitution and delegation within primary care.

Research approach and methods

The approach taken was broadly anthropological insofar as it was concerned to explore ideas, values and beliefs to which primary care professionals appeal in order to justify their work and distinguish it from the work of others. Since one way of understanding the culture of a profession (while acknowledging that it is not the only way) is to look at its written record, we undertook an intensive, systematic and detailed literature review. We also wanted to get a contemporary and critical perspective on issues raised in the literature, and so we arranged interviews with a total of fifteen commentators on both medicine and nursing. Data collection took place between September 1996 and January 1997.

Literature review methods

We drew on literature from several disciplines, mainly nursing and medicine, but also medical sociology and health services research, in part because nurses and doctors contribute to these literatures. The literature review was conducted using the following two main methods: (1) electronic literature searches (Medline, Bath Information and Data Services [BIDS], Cumulative Index of Nursing and Allied Literature [CINAHL]), using keywords derived from literature reviewed for the study proposal, and from sources derived from (2) a systematic exploration of journals, magazines, newspapers and bibliographies identified as relevant to the investigation. For example, throughout the study, current journals were surveyed in order to identify articles relating to study objectives. Key articles cited by the authors were, in turn, searched. As the study progressed, many articles were identified by interviewees. Some of these had already been reviewed by the researchers. Others were identified in this way. Thus, following Deeks *et al.* (1996), we aimed for comprehensiveness, and distinctions between research-based studies and commentary were noted.

Both methods proved fruitful but were not without their problems. Of the electronic sources accessed, Medline proved the most problematic, providing enormous databases and with most articles relevant to the USA. A further problem with most of the electronic searches was an apparent lack of sensitivity to the complexities and ambiguities of key study terms such as culture, change, environment, doctor–nurse interface, and loss and gain. Each of these key terms proved largely ineffective in the context of a Medline search, but each remained critical to the research.

The systematic search through journals and bibliographies challenged the researchers to discuss the sources most appropriate to the study, given that most articles in nursing and medical journals could be viewed as relevant in relation to a main study objective, namely to identify core ideas, values and beliefs in the respective professions. The method potentially creates a time-costly organizational problem. For example, almost any copy of a number of journals ranging from *Journal of Advanced Nursing* and *Advances in Nursing Science* to *Nursing Times* and *Nursing Standard* could be seen as relevant to an understanding of the scope and complexity of nursing.

The interviews

The purpose of the interviews was to provide representatives from nursing (chiefly) and medicine with the opportunity to comment from a professional standpoint on issues raised by the literature. In order to allow respondents the opportunity to expand at length and in depth on issues, the interviews were conducted within a qualitative research framework (following Oakley 1980; Finch 1984; Hammersley and Atkinson 1995). A qualitative framework allows for flexibility in the way the questions are formulated and in the sequencing of questions.

People were selected for interview on the basis of two broad categories of criteria. The first category encompassed those in a position to expand on issues raised in the literature, in some cases as contributors to the literature. This category included senior nurses, a spokesperson for primary care medicine, a spokesperson for consumer views, and a commentator on the social context of health care. The second category included those managing or working with current skill mix changes within primary health care, specifically a nurse manager, three general practitioners, two practice nurses, two health visitors and a district nurse.

A total of fifteen people were interviewed. Nine were interviewed face-to-face, three by telephone, and a further three were interviewed together as a group at their place of work. Some people crossed the criteria categories outlined above. For example, some of those in the second category had contributed to the literature. All interviews but one were audiotaped (with the permission of the respondents) and took between 45 and 90 minutes, with the majority averaging one hour. People interviewed were asked to sign a consent form. Consent forms were sent out to the three people who were interviewed by telephone and were returned with signatures. On one occasion a tape recorder was not used (owing to a technical breakdown). The respondent signed a consent form, and the researcher made detailed notes of the interview.

The key interview questions were as follows:

- How far is it the case that work formerly undertaken by general practitioners is being undertaken by nurses?
- What do you think are the main areas in which work is moving from doctors to nurses in primary care?
- What kind of relationship is being developed between doctors and nurses in primary care?
- What is being lost and gained as a consequence of changes (for both doctors and nurses)?
- What do you think will remain distinctive about medicine and what will remain distinctive about nursing in the primary care context?
- What is the overall impact of the current changes and development of roles (general practitioner and nursing) on primary care?

The audiotaped interviews were transcribed and scrutinized as follows. Correspondence and divergence between the broad answers to the questions posed were noted. Key words indicative of ideas, values and beliefs about professional concerns and the theory and practice of primary care were highlighted in order to comment on culture and cultural differences. Literature sources considered immediately relevant to points raised by respondents were noted in the margins of the typescripts.

Analysis

A thematic analysis of both the literature and the interviews was undertaken with the emphasis on the elucidation of ideas rather than the production of data amenable to statistical analysis (Silverman 1994; Hammersley and Atkinson 1995). Throughout, we aimed to read our data as indicative of cultural differences between medicine and nursing in relation to shifting boundaries between and within the two professions. The thematic analysis was structured as follows. Three working hypotheses were constructed, based on a preliminary review of literature and on current and ongoing research in related areas within the NPCRDC. A first hypothesis was that there is a change in skill mix within the primary care sector, and nurses are increasingly substituting for doctors in some areas of work (Marsh and Dawes 1995; Richardson and Maynard 1995; West 1995; Sibbald 1996). A second hypothesis was that boundary changes associated with role substitution raise issues around dimensions of work which might be seen to be either lost or enhanced (Short 1995; Bradshaw 1996). A third hypothesis, based on the emerging analysis, was that boundary changes associated with role substitution engender uncertainty associated with tension between, on the one hand, an impulse for innovation and, on the other hand, a retreat into the protection of 'profession'.

The working hypotheses guided the development of the literature review and, as indicated above, helped the researchers to formulate the interview questions. They also provided the framework for conveying the discussion of findings in the Summary Report (Williams *et al.* 1997) and as such provided the point of departure for the chapters that follow.

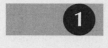 **Primary care: background and policy issues**

Bonnie Sibbald

The juxtaposition of medical and nursing cultures in primary care is nowhere more evident than in the general practice team. General practice is arguably the lynchpin of primary care, providing first contact, ongoing and comprehensive health care to people irrespective of their age, sex or presenting health problem. In the UK, the core general practice team since the 1990s has been typically composed of a partnership of three or four general medical practitioners which employs one or two practice nurses and an administrative staff composed largely of receptionists and secretaries (Usherwood *et al.* 1997). Other primary care professionals, notably district nurses, health visitors and midwives, work in close association with the practice to make up the 'extended' general practice team. The general practice therefore brings together one type of medical professional with a wide range of nursing professionals in a team jointly tasked with providing primary health care to a defined population.

To understand the cultural differences between nursing and medicine in primary care one must first understand the features which distinguish general medical practice from other medical specialities. This chapter deals with both these features and with the health policy pertaining to the organizational and contractual changes governing the general practitioner contract.

The origins of general medical practice

The cultural identity of general practice medicine has been shaped primarily by the need to differentiate it from and raise its status over other branches of medicine. Little attention has been paid to the boundaries with nursing because nursing has, until recently perhaps, never seriously challenged the identity or ethos of general practice.

General practitioners evolved from the apothecaries of medieval times whose chief competitors in health care provision included physicians and surgeons. Apothecaries were cheap, abundant, available to all members of the population and charged fees only for drugs. Physicians were the élite, charging high fees for their services and leaving the menial task of drug provision to the apothecaries. Surgeons occupied an intermediate position, being regarded as tradesmen like apothecaries, but enjoying a higher social status particularly during wartime. Physicians were the first to consolidate their status as professionals through the establishment in 1518 of the College of Physicians (later the Royal College of Physicians) which was granted the privilege to limit the practice of medicine to its licentiates, initially within London and later throughout England. The Company of Barber-Surgeons was granted similar privileges in 1629 with the foundation of the Royal College of Surgeons. In contrast, apothecaries were not distinguished from trades merchants by Royal Charter until 1617, and it was not until 1812 that the Society of Apothecaries received examining and licensing rights. Thus, as Oswald (1992) describes the situation in the eighteenth century,

> orthodox medical practitioners . . . were apparently rigidly divided into three groups: university-educated physicians who diagnosed but did not dispense and confined their activities to patients from the higher social classes; apothecaries who dispensed for themselves and for physicians, confining their diagnostic skill to the lower classes and pretending, for legal purposes, that it did not exist; and the surgeons, carrying on a trade involving the supervision of any external manifestation of disease or injury, or any procedure involving cutting of the skin.
>
> (p. 17)

These rigid distinctions were, however, difficult to maintain outside big conurbations such as London, with its large numbers of affluent people. Areas of low population density simply did not have the resources to sustain a tripartite system and competition among practitioners forced many to practise 'generally', that is across all three areas, in order to survive. Indeed this blurring of roles due to economic forces persisted well into the twentieth century and was only truly resolved with the introduction of the National Health Service in 1948 (Oswald 1992).

Legally, the apothecaries who wished to be accredited to do more than provide drugs were required to be licensed by one or the other of the Royal College of Physicians or Royal College of Surgeons. Each College evolved a 'second division' qualification specifically for this purpose, thus underlining the lower status of physician/surgeon apothecary. The term 'general practitioner' probably emerged early in the nineteenth century and was applied mainly to surgeon apothecaries who were both members of the Royal College of Surgeons and licentiates of the Society of Apothecaries. General practice was not clearly differentiated from other branches of medicine until the introduction of the Medical Act 1858 which established a single governing body, the General Medical Council (GMC), with the power to set overall standards and remove the license to practise of any doctor. The GMC was initially controlled by the two Royal Colleges (of Physicians and Surgeons) who agreed in 1884 to approve a joint diploma aimed primarily at general practitioners. General practitioners gained in the sense that they had succeeded in formally uniting their discipline, but at the price of occupying the lowest tier in the medical hierarchy (Royal College of General Practitioners 1992a).

The rapid growth in medical science throughout the late nineteenth and early twentieth centuries made it increasingly difficult for any one doctor to be familiar with all relevant knowledge and so led to the emergence of specialists. Specialization went hand in glove with the development of hospital medicine and the emergence of teaching hospitals as centres of excellence in teaching and research. This trend left general practitioners with an apparently diminishing role as mere gatekeepers to a hospital élite. The introduction of the National Health Service in 1948 did little to reverse this situation. While it established general practitioners as the principal providers of primary care, it also institutionalized their role as gatekeepers to secondary, specialist care. Prior to this time it was possible for general practitioners as well as physicians to act as specialist consultants in addition to providing general medical services. After the foundation of the National Health Service a clear line was drawn between general practitioners and consultant physicians. The former were restricted to providing general medical services in the community. This, in time, resulted in 'a narrowing of general practitioners' skills which was important in diminishing the status of general practice in the view of patients, specialists, and practitioners themselves' (Oswald 1992). General practitioners were sorely in need of a more positive professional identity, one which affirmed the unique knowledge base and skills of the general practitioner and gave 'generalism' the same status as specialism (Royal College of General Practitioners 1992b).

Such an identity was forged in a remarkably short period of time by a number of key thinkers and leaders in the field. William Pickles, a single-handed general practitioner in Yorkshire, received critical acclaim for his work on the spread of infectious diseases within his practice population, so demonstrating that general practitioners were capable of outstanding research without reference to hospitals and their resources. Other key figures included John Hunt and Fraser Rose, co-founders of the Royal College of General Practitioners in 1952, who were influential in drawing attention to the unique nature of general practice. Among the defining features were the centrality of the doctor/patient relationship in promoting health and the very different nature of the 'clinical material' from that seen in wards and outpatient departments. General practitioners were presented as experts in their field, on a par with specialists in other disciplines. These ideas fuelled a burgeoning body of research into general practice medicine which firmly established the unique knowledge base of the discipline (Royal College of General Practitioners 1992b). The rising status of general practice medicine was further consolidated in the 1970s and 1980s through the establishment in most medical schools of academic departments of general practice, and in the 1990s by successive government policies favouring a primary care-led National Health Service.

Despite these considerable achievements, general practice is still struggling to shake off its historical image as the discipline pursued by those who cannot make the grade in more prestigious medical specialities. General practitioners constitute 50 per cent of the UK medical workforce but fewer than 20 per cent of medical graduates positively opt for a career in general practice (Health Policy and Economic Research Unit 1998). There are fewer general practitioners with higher degrees than in all other medical specialities combined, and collectively general practitioners attract less than 5 per cent of all medical research funding (National Health Service Executive 1997a). Many of these problems arise historically from the different career structures and remuneration systems which encourage and reward specialists in hospital-based disciplines, but not primary care, to conduct research and develop higher professional skills. Understandably, general practice leaders remain focused on attaining equality of opportunity and status for their discipline relative to other medical specialities.

If the cultural identity of general practice medicine has been forged in relation to other medical specialities, the cultural identity of general practice nursing has arguably been forged in relation to medicine. Do nurses work independently and autonomously, or are they the handmaidens of the doctor? If nurses take on the work formerly carried out by doctors, do they lose their distinctive qualities as nurses? What are the cultural features which distinguish nursing from medicine? These are questions which attract considerable attention within the nursing, but not the medical, community (see, for example, Anonymous 1996; Atkin and Lunt 1996). The focus for debate within each profession is surely centred on points of vulnerability. General practice has struggled to carve its identity within medicine. Nursing has struggled to differentiate itself from medicine.

The nature of general medical practice

The defining features of general practice medicine deserve closer examination. Central themes in definitions of the role of the general practitioner include: personal, primary and continuing medical care to individuals and families; diagnoses framed in physical, psychological and social/contextual terms; educational, preventive and therapeutic interventions used to promote health; and the importance of the doctor/patient relationship as the medium for care delivery (Royal College of General Practitioners 1996).

Great importance is attached to seeing the patient and their illness in holistic terms and to healing as much as curing. So, for example, McWhinney, quoted by the Royal College of General Practitioners (1996) in its statement *The Nature of General Medical Practice* draws attention to the need for family doctors to frame assessments in terms of: clinical diagnosis (which is usually biomedical in orientation), individual diagnosis (which describes hopes, fears, feelings and expectations in relation to the problem) and contextual diagnosis (which describes the social or structural features of relevance). The College goes on to say that:

> Clinical diagnosis is the traditional scientific process, whereas individual diagnosis involves identifying the patient's perception of the problem and its possible causes. This is a highly personal process that is relevant to healing but often ignored by practitioners of scientific medicine. Contextual diagnosis reflects skilled awareness that many experiences of illness are re-inforced or perpetuated by social or family context, and healing is unlikely to be achieved if the wider issues remain unacknowledged or ill-considered.
>
> (Royal College of General Practitioners 1996: 2–3)

Two points of importance emerge from this statement. The first is that general practice is drawing attention to its difference from other medical specialities in the importance it attaches to individual and contextual factors in addition to more traditional biomedical factors in the practice of medicine. Secondly, in its emphasis on healing, not simply curing, general practice lays claim to one of the salient criteria which arguably distinguishes nursing from medicine. Nurses are often said to give more attention to caring than curing and so concentrate on 'social and emotional support and the creation of a therapeutic environment' (Ryan 1996). Much of the research on which such ideas have been founded, however, has referred to hospital settings, not primary care, and focused on nurse relations with physicians or surgeons, not general practitioners (see, for the example, the reviews of Sweet and Norman 1995; Ryan 1996). The situation may arguably be different in primary care settings given the different ethos of general practice medicine. Can it really be said that a district nurse managing leg ulcers among elderly patients in the community is less concerned about curing ulcers than with creating a therapeutic environment for patients? Does a nurse practitioner running a minor illness clinic in general practice not have as a main objective the resolution of those minor illnesses? Both caring and curing are central to the provision of primary health care which is characterized by the prevalence of undifferentiated illness which owes as much to the social and psychological context of people's lives as to their biomedical state. It is by emphasizing this aspect of care in community settings that general medical practice has sought to distinguish itself from hospital-based medicine – and perhaps unwittingly aligned itself with nursing.

Whether such attributes as holism, caring and curing genuinely distinguish patient/professional relationships in different branches of medicine or between nursing and medicine is highly contestable. What is perhaps more relevant is that professional groups have chosen to characterize themselves in these different ways. To the extent that the 'defining' attributes of a profession have clarity and meaning for its professionals, they frame the potential for future role development. Changes in the organization and delivery of care which challenge the defining features of the profession may be resisted, while those which are consistent with the ethos of the profession may be supported.

Delegation and skill substitution

Other key features of general practice medicine in the UK arise from the way the health care system is organized and therefore, unlike the attributes above, may differ from country to country. The UK has a primary care-centred health system. Primary care-centred health care systems have four key characteristics which arguably enhance the quality and cost-effectiveness of care as compared with other health care systems (Starfield 1992). These key characteristics include first contact care, longitudinality, comprehensiveness, and coordination. Primary care physicians are the main source of first contact care for new problems, ongoing care for long-term problems, and for preventive care and health promotion. Longitudinality means the primary care physician has a continuing relationship with the patient, potentially over a whole lifetime, encompassing different illnesses and episodes of care. Comprehensiveness means that the primary care physician undertakes responsibility for all health problems in populations except those that arise too uncommonly for the practitioner to maintain competence in dealing with them. The fourth key function is coordination of all aspects of care that are provided within primary care settings with those provided elsewhere.

These attributes are as integral to general medical practice in the UK as the more generic properties of the general practitioner described above. They clearly distinguish the role of the general practitioner from that of other medical providers and offer an evidence-based argument for the superior cost-effectiveness of a health care system which places primary care physicians to the fore. Fragmentation of the generalist role of the primary care physician among other health care providers or through the introduction of specialists into the primary care team, be they nurses, doctors, or others, threatens in theory the efficiency and cost-effectiveness of care. General practitioners have generally not been reluctant to *delegate* care to other health professionals, principally practice nurses, who are employed and supervised by them because they retain central responsibility for the care provided. In essence, the nurse extends the general practitioners' capacity in those areas which the doctor deems appropriate. Certainly, practice nurses in the 1990s have gained responsibility for much of the health promotion and chronic disease follow-up work of UK general practice (Ross *et al.* 1994; Bowling and Stilwell 1996). Some general practitioners, however, have regretted even this level of role fragmentation as it deprives them of the opportunity to care holistically for patients in the sense of dealing with all primary care problems.

The *substitution* of doctors by nurses in which doctors' responsibilities for patient care are transferred to autonomous professionals is another matter. Skill substitution clearly challenges the generalist role of the primary care physician. The issue here is often portrayed as one of power and control – more explicitly, one of powerful doctors' reluctance to surrender control to less powerful nursing and other professions. While there is undoubted truth in this, there is a more fundamental issue at stake. Will the substitution of nurses for doctors enhance the quality or cost-effectiveness of care? Research in this area is far from conclusive. The most substantive body of evidence is American in origin and has yet to be replicated within the very different health care system of the UK (Office of Technology Assessment 1986; Gibbs *et al.* 1991; Hopkins *et al.* 1996). There is no fundamental reason, however, why an appropriately trained nurse might not provide as good a service as a general practitioner. The question is really one of appropriate training and the acceptability to patients of nurse/doctor substitution. Properly managed skill substitution appears to pose few problems for patients (Office of Technology Assessment 1986; Stilwell 1996b). What constitutes appropriate training is debatable and it has been suggested that many nurses undertaking extended roles in general practice may be insufficiently qualified (see, for example, Bentley 1991; Ross *et al.* 1994). The problem, where it exists, can be rectified simply enough through the provision of additional training – always assuming that agreement can be reached on the standards to be attained. Taken to its logical extreme, the full substitution of doctors by nurses would imply that nurses should be retrained as doctors. This absurd conclusion might yet prove a reality if no clear understanding is reached about the purpose of skill substitution and its impact on patient health care.

To extend a point made in the introduction to this book, nurse/doctor substitution in UK primary care in the 1990s is said to be fuelled by: rising demand and cost of care which has increased interest in the possible economies to be made by shifting care from expensive to cheaper health professionals (Richardson and Maynard 1995); National Health Service policy changes which encourage a shift from hospital-based to community-based care, thereby increasing the volume and range of services demanded of primary care professionals (Department of Health 1996b); anticipated falls in the effective size of the general practitioner workforce consequent on a recent decline in recruitment to the speciality (Carlisle and Johnstone 1996; Lambert *et al.* 1996) and a move towards part-time working accentuated by the increasing proportion of female doctors (Taylor and Leese 1997). This is apart from any consideration that the different professions may be self-interestedly seeking to alter or extend their roles and influence.

A fundamental issue which has yet to be addressed is the overall impact of skill substitution on the quality and cost-effectiveness of primary health care delivery. Most research and commentary in the area of skill substitution has focused on restricted areas of care, for example nurse/doctor substitution in health promotion, diabetes care, asthma care, hypertension clinics and so on. No research has yet grappled with the wider problem of assessing how fragmentation of the generalist role of the general practitioner might impact on the overall quality and cost of service provision. International health systems analysts, such as Starfield (1992), have argued persuasively that the role of the generalist primary health care physician is a key factor in the superior cost-effectiveness of primary care-centred health care systems. It is therefore legitimate to question the wisdom of encouraging nurse/doctor substitution or indeed specialization by 'generalists' in either professional group in primary care.

Viewed from the perspective of the professionals themselves, the issue of whether it is doctors, nurses, or third parties who are controlling the direction of skill mix changes in general practice and primary care becomes less relevant when one is clear where one wants to be. Favourable directions of travel can be supported, and unfavourable ones opposed, irrespective of the agent(s) promoting the change or their motivations. In this sense, general practitioners as a group would appear to be on more secure ground than primary health care nurses – albeit the difference may be no more than standing on shifting sands as opposed to foundering in the sea. The professional bodies representing general practitioners are at least clear that they wish the profession to remain generalist primary care physicians (as described above). The professional bodies representing nursing, however, are uncertain whether it is consistent with the role of the nurse to extend her role into areas previously the province of doctors or alternatively work as a 'handmaiden' to the general practitioner. The dispassionate observer might argue that skill substitution should be encouraged if it enhances the efficiency or cost-effectiveness of health care provision.

Health care policy

Relationships between general practitioners and primary health care nurses have been much influenced by the organization of care within the National Health Service and by successive policy and contractual changes governing the general practitioner contract.

When the National Health Service was founded in 1948, general practitioners, unlike other doctors remained outside emergent health care organizations as *independent contractors*. In essence, they remained self-employed health care providers who contracted to provide an agreed package of *general medical services* to the National Health Service. Independent contractor status was, and is, seen by most general practitioners as a means of safeguarding their professional freedom and autonomy. Others have argued, however, that independent contractor status is principally a vehicle for fostering the professional status and ethos of the profession – initially when threatened by powerful, hospital-based medical specialities and, more recently, by government attempts to direct their work (Lewis 1997). Certainly it is true that general practice negotiators have consciously sought to ensure that successive contracts reflected the ideals and values of general practice as expressed by its professional bodies. It is also true, in common with other professional groups, that they have opposed attempts by outside agencies, notably government, to exercise authority over the quality and content of practice, reserving these rights to their own professional governing bodies.

Prior to the 1960s, general practitioners tended to work alone or in small partnerships of one or two doctors, unsupported by other clinical staff. The district nurse, midwife and health visitor generally worked independently of the general practice, serving a geographically defined population (commonly known as the patch or neighbourhood system). Relationships between general practitioners and community nurses were generally poorly developed, with little effective collaboration in care provision – which apparently suited the nursing and medical professionals alike. Concerns had been expressed, however, about the quality of primary care provision and, in 1963, the Standing Medical Advisory Committee of the Central Health Services Council recommended that improvements might be secured if 'fieldworkers' such as the nurse, midwife and health visitor were attached to individual practices (Standing Medical Advisory Committee and Standing Nursing and Midwifery Advisory Committee 1981). The debate about whether patch systems offered higher standards of care than attachment systems then raged for more than a decade. General practitioners favoured attachment systems because it allowed them better to coordinate care for their registered patients. Nurses were generally opposed to attachment systems as it reduced both their autonomy and their ability to care for the vulnerable members of a community who might not always be registered with a general practice.

General practitioners were able largely to circumvent the problems of securing nursing assistance in the practice with the introduction of the 1966 general practice contract. This enabled general practitioners to delegate work to nurses and to be reimbursed 70 per cent of the salary of nurses employed by the practice. Further legal changes were introduced in 1968 which permitted nurses employed by the health authority to extend their services from patients' homes to general practice surgeries and clinics. The contractual infrastructure was thus in place to permit growth in general practice 'teams' (Bowling and Stilwell 1996).

Teams were, however, slow to develop at least partly because general practitioners lacked the premises and financial resources needed to support larger teams. This situation gradually improved throughout the 1970s and 1980s as general practitioners came together in larger partnerships with commensurately larger premises, and local health authorities built health centres able to house extended general practice teams. By the early 1980s, more than 70 per cent of general practitioners were working in partnerships of three or more doctors; more than 25 per cent were located in health centres; and around 70 per cent of community nurses were attached to general practice surgeries. Indeed, the trend towards larger team size has continued unabated. From 1986 to 1996 the number of general practitioners in partnerships of more than six increased by two-thirds; there was a fivefold increase in practice nurses; and administrative staff doubled in number (Health Policy and Economic Research Unit 1996).

The early development of teams was also checked by a growing policy debate in the 1980s on the advisability of allowing general practitioners to coordinate the work of attached nurses, let alone employ nurses themselves. The Cumberlege Report of 1986 (Department of Health and Social Security 1986a) condemned the remuneration system which allowed general practitioners to be 'paid twice' for work carried out by nurses in their employ – firstly in terms of fee-for-service and secondly through 70 per cent reimbursement of the nurse's salary. Cumberlege saw it as more appropriate that practice nurses be employed within health authority nursing teams where their training and development might be more closely supervised and their services better integrated with those of other community nurses in a patch-based system. These ideas were in direct opposition to the government's own policy on primary care, published at the same time, which advocated continuation of the remuneration system for practice-employed nurses (Department of Health and Social Security 1986b). The General Medical Services Committee, representing general practice interests, also retaliated strongly against the Cumberlege proposals (General Medical Services Committee 1986). The Royal College of Nursing, while sympathetic to the recommendations, did not feel able to support changes which threatened the jobs of so many of its constituents (Bowling and Stilwell 1996). The views of the medical lobby eventually prevailed. The general practitioners' right to employ nurses and, where appropriate, be reimbursed a proportion of their salary costs, has since been upheld in successive general practitioner contracts.

The question of whether health authority employed community nurses should be attached to general practices had reached no clear resolution, when the introduction of general practitioner fundholding in the early 1990s completely altered the balance of power in general practitioners' favour. As part of the initiative to foster an internal market in the National Health Service, fundholding general practices were enabled to purchase community nursing services from newly created NHS trusts (NHS Management Executive 1993). Most fundholders exercised this opportunity in ways which ensured that community nurses were attached to practices and worked in a more integrated way with practice-employed nurses. The traditional professional boundaries and networks among and between different types of community nurse were actively challenged (Atkin and Lunt 1996; Hiscock and Pearson 1996) in the effort to remove 'frustrating constraints' (Irvine 1993) and so achieve a more flexible, more responsive workforce. Health visitors, among the most expensive of community nurses and with a strong tradition of autonomous working, fared least well, as general practitioners saw many of their services as either redundant or more appropriately and cheaply provided by others. Boundaries between practice nurses and district nurses were eroded in order to deploy individual nurses where their skills might most effectively be utilized. So, for example, district nurses were encouraged to undertake more extended roles in health provision within general practice clinics, while practice nurses visited patients at home to carry out health promotion assessments and check-ups.

The structure of primary health care provision in the UK and successive health policy developments have therefore given general practitioners greater control than nurses over the development of primary health care nursing services. As employers or 'purchasers', general practitioners have been better able than community nurses to promulgate their values and ideals. This is not to say that general practitioners have had it all their own way. The introduction of an internal market in the National Health Service in 1990 created an enormous administrative burden for practices, particularly those which opted to become fundholding. Many general practitioners complained that this increased administrative workload considerably reduced the time they could make available to patient care (Myerson 1992). An additional concern was the increased role that general practitioners were asked to play in public health and health services commissioning. In essence this placed general practitioners in the position of 'rationing' services – an activity which many believed conflicted with their role as personal care physicians and patients' advocates (Royal College of General Practitioners 1996). A final concern was the burden placed on practices by the drive to shift services from hospitals into primary care. General practitioners considered that insufficient attention was paid to the training and resource implications of shifting services and were concerned about the lack of additional remuneration for undertaking this new work (General Medical Services Committee 1996a). These concerns are important in that they will continue to shape general practitioners' response to the health service reforms set out in 1997.

Future developments

A change in government in 1997 saw the abolition of an internal market in the National Health Service and the introduction of new management systems based on more collaborative ways of working (Department of Health 1998). In respect of primary health care services, the government proposed the establishment of primary care groups (PCGs) and their equivalents (for example, local health groups [LHGs] in Wales) which would gradually take over from health authorities the task of commissioning health services for defined populations of approximately 100,000 people. Primary care groups are to be governed by a board composed of between four and seven general practitioners, one or two community or practice nurses, one social service officer nominee, one lay member, one health authority non-executive and one primary care group chief officer/manager (National Health Service Executive 1998). Local general practitioners have the right, but not the obligation, to be in a majority on the board and to have a general practitioner as chair of the board. Primary care groups will have responsibility for developing and implementing a health implementation plan to meet the health care needs of their local population, managing health care expenditure and assuring the quality of health care delivery. The intention is that these groups will eventually evolve into autonomous primary care trusts with responsibility for both providing and commissioning primary health care services. Many expect that primary care trusts will be formed through the merger of community health care trusts with local consortia of general practices.

At one level these proposals would appear to reinforce the position which general practitioners have enjoyed in shaping the health care agenda in primary care. They are clearly being offered the opportunity to assume the leading role in the management and development of primary health care services. Some will seize upon this opportunity, notably those who were previously in the forefront of general practitioner fundholding and total purchasing initiatives. However, closer examination reveals an underlying agenda for change which in a number of respects may challenge the traditional ethos and power of general practitioners.

The most obvious difficulty lies in making general practitioners explicitly responsible for the allocation of health spending within a locality. While some general practitioners have welcomed this opportunity, many more have expressed concern about being made publicly responsible for 'rationing' decisions within the National Health Service. As mentioned above, the Royal College of General Practitioners has voiced the opinion that the responsibility for commissioning health services on behalf of defined populations in many ways conflicts with the general practitioners' key role as a personal physician and patient advocate (Royal College of General Practitioners 1996). Many are additionally concerned about the added management and administrative burden for which they may not be fully remunerated. Only a minority of general practitioners may therefore be willing to take up the new responsibilities and opportunities afforded by these health service reforms.

An added consideration is that, as independent contractors, general practitioners have no tradition of working together within larger organizational structures and have strongly resisted attempts by previous governments to exercise greater control over the quality and content of their services. Primary care groups have explicit authority for 'clinical governance', that is for assuring standards of clinical care, and for ensuring that local health services adequately meet local health needs. If they are to discharge these functions successfully, they will need actively to coordinate and direct the work of local general practices and institute systems for monitoring quality. This challenges the notions of clinical autonomy and freedom which general practitioners have valued as independent contractors. Indeed, it is reasonable to suppose that the introduction of primary care groups and their evolution into primary care trusts, will lead to the phasing out of independent contractor status for general practitioners and bring them under the direct control of conventional National Health Service organizations. A number of associated policy changes are in place to facilitate this transition. For example, the government has sought to extend and develop the options for salaried service by general practitioners within the National Health Service. Policy changes in 1997 relaxed the conditions under which general practitioners could be employed by independent contractor colleagues and directed health authorities to give priority to encouraging uptake of these options (National Health Service Executive 1997b). Elsewhere, the Primary Care Act 1996, enabled the Secretary of State for Health to approve experimental sites whereby practices, not individual general practitioners, contract to provide general medical services. The same legislation has enabled nurse-led and community trust-led practices to be established. Eighty-eight such experimental sites were approved in 1998 and a further wave is planned. While these initiatives have yet to be fully evaluated, the expectation is that many general practitioners will find them highly attractive as they have the potential to free doctors from unwanted management responsibilities and offer greater flexibility in terms of clinical responsibility and hours of work. The next few years will be crucial in determining whether an increasing majority of general practitioners feel that the benefits of salaried employment within new National Health Service organizations outweigh those of independent contractor status.

It is far from certain, therefore, that the primary care organizations of the future will be run by general practitioners. Indeed, it is possible that general practitioners, like nurses and other health practitioners, will be employed within a National Health Service organization run by professional managers. From a structural point of view, there is no reason to suppose that such organizations will give greater weight to the voices of doctors over nurses, although the longstanding issues of medical dominance and the sexual division of labour may serve to perpetuate the dominance of doctors. The insistence by successive governments on greater public accountability within the health services makes it most likely that both groups will see their future role development governed by forces outside the health professions altogether. Should general practitioners continue to be preoccupied with their status *vis-à-vis* other medical specialities and should nurses continue to be preoccupied with their boundary with medicine, both will easily be manipulated by those concerned only with improving the efficiency and cost-effectiveness of the National Health Service for the greater good of the people.

2 Boundary changes in primary care

As noted in Chapter 1, the shape and ethos of an emerging primary care within the UK owes much to the efforts of general practice medicine to distinguish itself from hospital medicine. However, recent pressure to improve the cost-effectiveness of primary care through role substitution and the strategic delegation of areas of care from expensive to cheaper health care providers (Marsh and Dawes 1995; Richardson and Maynard 1995; West 1995; Sibbald 1996) draws our attention to the boundary between medicine and nursing, the focus for discussion in this chapter.

The chapter commences by returning to the term 'substitution' in the context of health care, taking into account the ambiguity which it appears to invite – ambiguity made evident in the various ways in which the term is interpreted. Discussion moves on to consider the ways in which the impetus for current boundary changes between medicine and nursing is analysed and understood. Three areas of analysis are identified in this respect: medical control, ascendancy of nursing arguments, and economic concerns. Throughout the chapter, account is taken of the historical relationship between the two professions and also the changing contemporary scene where, despite the recent calls for flexibility and interprofessional collaboration (Department of Health 1998; Welsh Office 1998a), the legacy of professional affiliation remains strong.

'Substitution'

The word 'substitution', when used to describe the process by which work moves from doctors to nurses, carries a number of possible meanings. From a health services perspective, substitution is associated with broadly economic concerns about the redistribution of work to increase efficiency, effectiveness and consumers' satisfaction (Richardson and Maynard 1995). The economics of care is by now a matter of concern for all health professionals;

however, the use of the word 'substitution' in nursing and medicine also displays interests and beliefs which touch on professional identity and purpose. As the following discussion suggests, there are substantial differences between primary care medicine and nursing in this respect.

A medical perspective and its antecedents

It becomes apparent that when some general practitioners use the word 'substitution' they mean delegation, or the implementation of 'prescribed' work. This view is reflected by, for example, Stern (1996), Rashid et al. (1996) and Lenehan and Watts (1994), the latter in relation to practice nurses, but not in relation to nurse practitioners. An underlying assumption is that nurses follow doctors' orders which, as Mackay (1993) reports, was a view widely held by doctors in her extensive survey-based enquiry into interprofessional relations between doctors and nurses. This is not to say that general practitioners intentionally treat nursing as the 'handmaiden' of medicine rather than as a separate role. Indeed, they might strenuously deny so and, in many individual instances, general practitioners support attempts by nurses to improve their position through further education and training, a point reiterated throughout the book. Nevertheless, medicine's status in relation to nursing has been evident in policies promoting the leadership of general practice medicine in primary care since 1948, and it is implicit in individual commentary by well-meaning general practitioners who appear to be working with 'their' nurses towards an integrated approach (Richardson 1997), collaboration (Strachan 1997) and contract negotiations with trusts (Smith 1996).

Perhaps we should not be surprised. The difference in status between medicine and nursing has been a topic of sociological debate over the years. There are two broad planks upon which the debate rests: first, analyses of the overall societal hierarchy in which professions in general are located and second, analyses of dimensions of the relationship between the two professions.

In brief, analyses of the overall societal hierarchy within which professions are located draw on ideas about inequalities in power and status in order to illuminate an understanding of the relationship between professional groups. Class and capitalism are wider forms of social structure and inequality; however, as Walby et al. (1994) suggest (following others), reliance on these forms for an understanding of professions is insufficient as they ignore the gendered structure of society. The authors stress that the latter is important especially when considering the relationship between the largely male-dominated profession of medicine and the largely female-dominated profession of nursing. The issue of sex is theorized in the following ways: at a social psychological level where sex attributes are seen as a result of socialization, and at a structural level where sex is produced as a result of structures including the family, state and labour market. The former sees occupation and behaviour within it as a matter of choice on the basis of an individual's values, while in the latter theory the position of the occupation within employment hierarchies is seen as the result of structures of power relations. Indeed, the lowly position of nurses compared with doctors is related to the wider position of women in society, the causal links including women's lesser formal political power (Walby *et al*. 1994: 64).

Ideas about power and status also dominate discussions of professional relationships between doctors and nurses in health care settings. Davies (1980), and Witz (1992) suggest that professionalization for nurses has been partial because of sustained medical control over key aspects of nursing. Stacey (1988) notes how medical men had from the outset established themselves in a powerful position and ensured the subservience of nurses and midwives. 'Subordination' and 'subservience' are words which have come to characterize analyses of nursing's relationship with medicine. Porter (1995) in his study of doctor/nurse relationships in the acute care sector identifies a number of types of interaction that have been posited: unmitigated subordination whereby the nurses carry out doctors' orders without question; the pretence of unmitigated subordination as noted by Stein (1978), whereby nurses are deferential to doctors and refrain from open disagreement while at the same time attempting to have some input into the decision-making process; and informal overt decision making, a type of interaction noted by Hughes (1988) whereby intervention by nurses into decision making is open and deliberate but does not enjoy any official sanction. Porter explored nurses' views on these types of interaction and the extent to which they saw them as relevant to their own interactions with doctors. Unmitigated subordination was considered to be rare; informal covert decision making appeared to be a widely practised nursing strategy, whereas informal overt decision making was under-used.

Analyses of professions and professionalization which focus on power provide a critique of earlier analyses (Vollmer and Mills 1966) which viewed professions in terms of essential characteristics or traits. Distinctive professional traits varied on several dimensions: a distinctive knowledge base, the notion of altruistic service, and a profession's commitment to self-monitoring of professional activities and its own methods of training and assessment of competence. Walby and her colleagues (1994) indicate (the issue of power notwithstanding) that there may be some merit to the latter analysis insofar as it highlights the special relationship between knowledge and forms of occupational control possessed by professions.

A nursing perspective

While there is no doubt that medicine has had an important role in structuring its neighbouring occupations, especially nursing (Larkin 1983), there is an increasing resistance to medical interference in nursing education and practice. Nurses have sought to construct a professional identity which sets nursing apart from medicine and which does not restrict nurses to the biomedical model of care. Thus nurses draw on social psychology and psychotherapy disciplines which emphasize meaningful interaction between nurse and patient (Salvage 1992). The profession also draws on sociology and social policy which increase a critical awareness of nursing's position in contemporary society and the scope of its professional project. In addition, the United Kingdom Central Council (UKCC) Code of Conduct and related documents was significantly revised in 1992 in order to provide a basis for independent, professional judgement where principles for practice replace certificates for tasks (UKCC 1992a, b, c). This marks a move in UK nursing from a rule-focused approach to one of individual judgement. Together with efforts by the Council of Deans of Nursing Midwifery and Health Visiting and the UKCC's Commission on Nurse Education – both of which press the advantages of moving nursing education into the higher education sector – it reflects the wider move in Europe and in the USA to produce degree-level nurses who are confident collaborators and who are prepared to be accountable for the care they deliver.

In recent years, the growing sense of professional identity and increasing awareness of the possibility of a distinctive contribution to health care means that for some nurses, the word 'substitution' tends to be associated with a sense of diminished status within nursing as is suggested in the question, 'are nurse practitioners *merely* substitute doctors?' (Anon 1996, emphasis added) and the following statement: 'the UKCC has been told that the work of nurse practitioners cannot be described as advanced as many are *only* doctor substitutes' (Mathieson 1996, emphasis added). Nurse commentators appear to prefer the word 'expansion' to substitution, noting that the former is a term to be distinguished from ideas about role extension (Zarnow 1977; Wright 1995). Nurses also refer to the '"transformation" of nursing roles, responsibilities and functions' (Bailey 1996). They construe new work and responsibilities as a 'complementary service which increases patient choice . . . enhances collaboration with the nursing profession, and enhances the scope of the skill mix across the primary health care team' (Anon 1996: 326).

In summary, the word 'substitution' can be quite revealing about how nurses identify themselves as different from doctors, and vice versa, in relation to work which moves from the latter to the former. That nurses are substituting for doctors in some areas of work is a statement that can be read as a fact, and areas of work can be usefully listed to give a sense of the scope of boundary changes in primary care work. However, interpretations of the process of substitution also convey a sense of the assumptions, aspirations and beliefs which accompany change and the ideas and values to which groups appeal in order to justify their work and to differentiate it from the work of others. In the following discussion both readings are applied to the literature and to the empirical study data in order to explore the ways in which the impetus for current boundary changes between medicine and nursing is analysed and understood.

Analyses of the impetus for boundary changes

Nurses, together with colleagues in medicine, the social sciences and health services research broadly agree that the impulse for boundary changes between nursing and medicine hinges primarily on number of key, related factors: the health system, the role of doctors and the economics of care (cf. Stilwell 1996a). The nature of the impact of these factors is accounted for in different and sometimes contradictory ways. For example, the growth in general practice fundholding in the early 1990s was seen as increasing general practitioners' power to shape the nature and organization of primary care nursing. Paradoxically, the introduction of the market was also seen as a destabilizing force with the potential to increase opportunities for nurses who were seeking to extend and expand their roles within primary care. The change of government in 1997 brought about the end of fundholding; however, general practitioners have maintained their leading role in primary care by virtue of their right to be in a majority in primary care groups (PCGs) in England, local health groups (LHGs) in Wales and their equivalents. Recent White Papers (National Health Service 1998; Welsh Office 1998a) emphasize collaboration and a duty of partnership, while at the same time there is a suggestion that competition is unlikely to disappear given the government's concern to retain aspects of the internal market that have worked (National Health Service 1998). Throughout the debates about the impetus for change, there is strong recognition of government pressure to improve the cost-effectiveness of primary care provision.

The remainder of this chapter outlines three broad areas of analysis where the factors identified above intersect. They are: medical control, ascendancy of nursing arguments, and economic concerns.

Medical control: licence and limitations

From both medical and health services research perspectives, it has been suggested that the internal market introduced by the Conservative administration in the 1989 White Paper *Working for Patients* (Department of Health 1989) greatly increased general practitioners' power to shape the nature and organization of community nursing services. General practice fundholding and general practice-influenced purchasing of community nursing services generally encouraged a breakdown in the boundaries between health visitors, district nurses and practice nurses to achieve greater flexibility in the deployment of nurse skills (Richardson and Maynard 1995). General practitioners contracted both to bring health visitors into practices to manage their health promotion services and to remove the boundaries between district nurses and practice nurses, encouraging the former to undertake 'delegated' medical tasks within practices and the latter to provide nursing care in the home. In her review of research and policy, Ridsdale (1993) has commented that nurses have increasingly undertaken medical tasks delegated by the general practitioner and they work under the day-to-day clinical direction of doctors rather than senior nurses.

Commentary from respondents who participated in the NPCRDC study suggests that in some cases this aspect of the process of boundary change has not been straightforward. For example, nurses we spoke to who were attached to a general practice felt that being attached rather than being directly employed by a practice offered them some protection against general practitioner control. This is how one health visitor described the situation in 1996 in the practice to which she was attached: 'I think we would probably have some concerns at being directly employed by GPs because they would then be able to dictate what we do . . . They'd want control. At the moment it's more about who they want to do the job – the grade – not what we actually do'. Her colleague added that the general practitioners wanted to see more overlap between district nurses and practice nurses, noting that 'they are not pushing but this is the mood'. This observation was followed by an obtuse comment suggesting that 'while the GPs would like to see more overlap it could be that they, the GPs, would never actually do anything about it'. When prompted, she replied, 'because I don't think they really know what they could do about it'.

The health visitor's words can be read as a suggestion that the nurses who, in this instance, were attached to a practice, as opposed to being employed, still felt an element of control over their work. Given that the words were spoken during a time of speculation about an immediately forthcoming government White Paper, *Choice and Opportunity* (Department of Health 1996a), they could also be read as an indication of the nurses' awareness of a degree of uncertainty on the part of general practitioners about future possibilities for nurses. From another perspective, the words 'they are not pushing [for overlap between district nurses and practice nurses] but this is the mood' reflect the nurse's awareness of the distinct possibility that boundaries between nurses could potentially break down, given the situation, then, of general practice fundholding and the primacy of general practitioners in future plans for primary care (Health Services Management Unit 1996; Salter and Snee 1997).

As indicated, medicine to date has been successful in securing power and status in health services provision within the UK. However, as Walby *et al.* (1994) point out, there are those who hold that medicine is losing power, becoming either 'proletarianized' or 'deprofessionalized'. Proletarianization here refers to the idea that medicine is now undergoing a transformation of its labour process equivalent to that described by Marx as affecting independent artisans in the Industrial Revolution who, through their incorporation into a factory production system, lost their autonomy and skills (Elston 1991: 63). The idea of proletarianization has been discussed mainly in relation to American medicine and it is alleged that US physicians face increasing economic, organizational and technical alienation from their labour. Elston writes:

> Alienation, and associated loss of autonomy and dominance, is attributed to the bureaucratisation of the American health care system, a process occurring through increasing state control of the financing of health care and increasing state control of health care for profit.
>
> (1991: 63)

It is suggested that even within a bureaucratized UK National Health Service, doctors have more clinical autonomy than their American counterparts but less economic autonomy. In the UK, the challenge to medicine's autonomy comes from the introduction of general management in the mid-1980s following the publication of the Griffiths Report in 1982 (Department of Health and Social Security 1983). Walby and colleagues write: 'the introduction of general management in the mid-1980s following the Griffiths Report is widely interpreted as one of the most significant attempts to curtail the power of the profession by managers in the history of the NHS' (Walby *et al.* 1994: 76). Central government introduced the first national set of National Health Service performance indicators (from 1983) and encouraged health authorities to experiment with management budgeting (Harrison and Pollitt 1995: 8). With the introduction of internal markets in 1989 (through the White Paper *Working for Patients*), the Conservatives sought to contain and redirect medical expenditure. Government's aim was to place management values within medical practice rather than to impose them from outside (Walby *et al.* 1994: 76). Doctors were to measure their own performance and cost, run their own budgets and compete with each other.

The deprofessionalization thesis is associated mainly with a decline in the cultural authority of medicine especially in relation to patients. The successful control of clients is seen by some theorists, notably Johnstone (1972), to be the critical distinguishing feature of professional power. Elston's (1991) analysis in respect of medicine is helpful. She outlines three strands of a potential challenge to medicine from the 'articulate consumer' (pp. 77–83). The first she describes as a cultural critique of interventionist medicine's ineffectiveness. This critique she explains, drawing on Starr (1982), is connected with a challenge to medicine's achievement of near-monopoly over the market for health care by the early twentieth century; the near-monopoly having been achieved through medicine's association with the values of science. Proponents of the critique challenged the beneficence of a medical science which produced thalidomide and other pharmacological disasters. A second strand is described by Elston as an aspect of the strongly individualistic element of the 1980s and early 1990s. This took the form of attacks on state legitimated licensed monopoly and a call for exposing state-sponsored activities to market forces, for example in general practice by increasing the sensitivity of general practitioners' pay to patient workload. The third strand can be summarized as the challenge from dissatisfied patients in respect of the inadequacies of institutionalized systems of victim compensation, the questioning of professional self-regulation and the implications for medical practice of increasing litigation (see Elston 1991 for a fuller discussion).

Both Elston and Walby *et al.* (1994) have noted a lack of hard evidence for the proletarianization and the deprofessionalization theses. The proletarianization thesis is criticized partly on the grounds that its proponents (McKinlay and Archer 1985; McKinlay and Stoeckle 1988) ignore sociological debates about the development of 'a service class' and the significance of educational credentials for class formation as discussed by Giddens (1973; see also Elston 1991: 63). The deprofessionalization thesis rests on ideas about the articulate consumer and the rise of information technology. Elston writing in 1991 comments on the lack of evidence to support the idea that greater computer use demystifies and routinizes medical procedures, making them more amenable to lay scrutiny (p. 64). Nearly a decade later, while it could be argued that computer use has transformed day-to-day living for those who have access and the technology promises benefits to the provision of health care, we find a consumerist challenge to medicine's authority still embryonic and it appears that many general practitioners are themselves struggling with information systems (Green *et al.* 1998). Despite criticisms, the proletarianization and deprofessionalization theses have been used to formulate the following argument for boundary changes between medicine and nursing, where nursing is seen to be in the ascendancy.

The ascendancy of nursing argument and its critics

In talking about the ascendancy of nursing argument, I do not mean to imply a strongly acknowledged argument with clearly identified protagonists. Rather, the term refers to a number of recent and in some ways rather *ad hoc* expressions, predominantly by nurses, of the opportunities for nurses to take on further responsibilities and to gain greater autonomy *vis-à-vis* medicine in a society which is rapidly changing. A recent example is provided by Kelly (1996) who suggests an analysis of boundary changes which acknowledges the role of external, socioeconomic forces in changing roles in primary care, but one which plays down the influence of medicine. She writes:

> Increasing state and corporate involvement in medical care and education, the bureaucratization of work organizations and decreasing public confidence are bringing changes in the market position of doctors.

Diminution of autonomy and influence over policy making are noted, and doctors are being relegated to the ranks of 'wage slaves': a process of proletarianization, and de-professionalization is occurring.

(Kelly 1996: 49)

This analysis in some respects echoes the work of Williams *et al.* (1993: 62) who raise questions about the possibility of declining general practitioner autonomy in the primary care sector, including the question of 'whether nurses will be able to extend their role and if so, will this represent a challenge to GP autonomy?' The authors do not arrive at a firm conclusion. Rather they underline how the 'frontiers of control' are in a state of uncertainty (p. 64). In some agreement with this position, a study respondent underlined the significance of collapsing class and sex boundaries in medicine, and the significance of the challenge, by society, to professionals in general, citing recent public challenges to scientists' knowledge about BSE (Bovine Spongiform Encephalopathy) and CJD (Creutzfeldt-Jakob Disease).

Kelly (1996: 49) asks the following questions. Is there a deliberate move to institute skill substitution? Can the ascendancy of the nursing profession be acceptable as a post-Fordist strategy to introduce reorganization of forms of health care delivery? Is there a political move to bring about the ascendancy of the nursing profession as an alternative to medical care? As readers will be aware, post-Fordism is to be distinguished from Fordism which is typified by large-scale, inflexible production of standardized products and refers to production which 'demands a different style of work organization. Workers require greater skill and they must be adaptable and willing to acquire new skills and knowledge' (Watson 1987: 96). The questions posed by Kelly can be read as hinting of theories about socioeconomic forces afoot to destabilize the professions (Crompton 1990; Fournier 1997), although, as Crompton (1996) notes, the patriarchal model of paid employment is difficult to dislodge.

Kelly's words can also be read as part of a nursing agenda to challenge medicine as and when opportunities arise. For example, Hancock (1997) writes:

The latest government white paper, *Delivering the Future*, maps out the long awaited ascendancy of nurses in delivering primary health care. It supports what the Royal College of Nursing has known for a long time – that if we are serious about building a primary care led NHS, we need to put nurses at its heart.

(p. 17)

Hancock elaborates:

Nurses have taken Bevan's vision and developed a health service which is more responsive to patients, which identifies communities' needs and promotes good health, as well as caring for people who are sick . . . Changes in primary care contracts outlined in the proposed Primary

Care Bill pave the way for nurses to become equal partners in general practice.

(p. 17)

Hancock's words 'partners in general practice' appear to relate, predominantly, to the nature of the clinical and professional relationship between medicine and nursing. 'Partnership' read in the sense of ownership, in financial terms, of the business was raised by some of our interviewees. One general practitioner commented that 'the future's for nurses' and gave the example of a nurse in the practice who would readily take on a partnership, although he thought that there may be deficits in the orientation of nurses for such a role. He observed:

> Nurses at the moment are subdividing and splitting up their role into specialisms as nurses at a time when general practitioners are emphasizing and developing their generalist roles. General practitioners see themselves . . . as a person who makes an initial decision. Whereas, nurses very often are saying, 'that's not for me, that's for the psychiatric nurse; that's not for me, that's for the stoma nurse, or the diabetic nurse.'

The general practitioner's words refer to a specialist pathway of nursing care provision which, in his view, the nurses are pursuing too far, and he posed the question: 'are they, in fact, impeding their development as a holistic visitor?' – a point revisited later in Chapter 3 (see p. 55).

A number of factors militate against arguments about the ascendancy of nursing. As Hiscock and Pearson (1996) point out in their case-study-based analysis of professional costs and invisible value in the community nursing market:

> Since GPs purchase *and* provide services, fundholding does not fit comfortably . . . with the recent emphasis on GPs working as colleagues in primary health care teams with primary and community healthcare nurses whom they may directly employ, or whose services they purchase.
> (Hiscock and Pearson 1996: 23–4)

This comment underlines the importance of taking existing power relations into account and counters any easy assumption that the nursing profession is in the ascendancy. It moderates assertions that the role of nursing is 'expanding' in the context of primary care. Indeed, Denner (1995), commenting on the new nursing roles, writes that nurse practitioners do little more than reinforce the traditional 'handmaiden' relationship with medicine. As one NPCRDC study respondent, a nurse, pointed out with reference to nurses across the primary/secondary sectors:

> nurses have always had a residual role, if there aren't enough doctors around, you're discovered! If there are, you get told to make tea . . . My perception is that nurses are being allowed in again, but I don't think it's through the rediscovery of the positive value of the nurse. I think

it's the discovery of the boundaries to the medical workforce in terms of its capacity. I'd like to think it was more positive. Sadly, I don't think it is . . .

Shepherd *et al.* (1996) take a similar line of argument. They give the example of nurse prescribing and extend Ridsdale's 1993 analysis, which is that nurses increasingly work under the day-to-day direction of general practitioners rather than nurses. They suggest that throughout the history of nursing and medicine, doctors have 'delegated' a range of duties which have become the defining features of nursing work. They write, 'such acts of "delegation" have become a one-way process and have reinforced the dominant position of medicine within the division of labour' (pp. 469–70). In respect to nurse prescribing, they underline the possibility of a reading of evidence which suggests that prescribing by community nurses can be considered in terms of acceptance of 'delegated' authority (p. 470). They note how the sites chosen for piloting UK nurse prescribing were ones in which there was clear budgetary control by the general practitioners.

Both Ridsdale (1993) and Shepherd *et al.* (1996) use the word 'delegation' implying the idea of transfer of work, rather than the word 'substitution' which, in contrast, implies mutuality and exchange of role. The use of the word 'delegation' is telling and suggests that despite moves to develop a sound and distinctive body of knowledge, nurses continue to face an uphill struggle against the power of medicine to define nursing roles and work (Soothill 1998: vii–viii).

Economic concerns

The context within which boundary changes are occurring is complex. Even if it were conceivable that external forces of deprofessionalization might prompt reorganization of forms of health care delivery such that the balance of power is altered between doctors and nurses, there remain the influential (if contested) issues of economy, namely efficiency and cost-effectiveness. Any danger to the development of the nurse's role, autonomy and potential influence in primary care is as likely to be a result of economic forces as it is to be an imbalance between the professional power of medicine versus nursing. In primary care the two are intimately related, given a situation where nurses are salaried and general practitioners are, at least at present, for the most part self-employed. When interviewed, one of our study respondents, a nurse, alluded to the economics of change in relation to nurses' work:

Round the country there's a whole lot of experiments going on . . . that give nurses the idea that . . . they are moving forward and it's all an exciting, challenging new world. And you're getting very naive, very inexperienced . . . nurses to think that they've only got to go into their own area of practice and develop something and the world will be their oyster and, you know, two years later, sadder and wiser, they discover that they've put in a lot of energy and hard work and nobody wants to keep it going . . . If they [nursing initiatives] don't prove to be enormous money savers, which inevitably they won't . . . they actually demand extra expenditure . . . rather than a cutback in existing expenditure . . . people lose interest – the managers.

The quotation encapsulates the dilemma experienced since the mid-1970s, not only by nurses but by a market-driven workforce in general. The dilemma is this: how to reconcile what appear to be opposing models of work and, relatedly, opposing sets of values. Harrison and Pollitt (1995) hint at the dilemma when, writing about health professionals, they comment on how 'the unrelenting emphasis on the desirability of market-like mechanisms has [had] considerable implications for professionals and managers alike. First it implies a . . . move away from the traditional model of lifetime professional carers, working under terms and conditions of service' (p. 12). The authors note that public service providers of the future will be working within contract or contract-like agreements which will be time limited and strictly costed.

The dilemma for health service workers such as nurses arises from a contradiction between the two models of work: on the one hand, a lifetime professional service carer and, on the other, time-limited and costed work. Underpinning this contradiction in models of work is a contradiction in values. As the quotation above illustrates, values of public service accompanied by the expectation that one has a working lifetime sit in uneasy juxtaposition with values of the market, notably what has come to be called enterprise culture – a phrase which, while it may have its origins in the competitive capitalism of past centuries, became highly politicized in the Thatcherite years when government reforms involved the extension of the domain of the free market to public institutions. This was accompanied by political rhetoric which gave prominence to the qualities of initiative, independence, self-reliance, a willingness to take risks and to accept responsibility for one's own actions (Keat and Abercrombie 1991: 3). There was a sense in which these enterprise qualities were seen as belonging to the Thatcherite agenda although, as Keat and Abercrombie and the contributors to their classic collection argue, Thatcherite enterprise was only one variant of enterprise culture. Enterprise is a generic category which could be 'utilized by more collectively oriented . . . socialist market systems' (Keat and Abercrombie 1991: 15). Indeed, we catch glimpses of this possibility in the recent government health reforms since the ascendancy of Labour in 1997. The dilemma remains for health care workers and there is no certainty that initiatives will 'pay off'.

Stilwell (1996a), a major contributor to research on initiatives in primary care nursing, notes how role substitution in the USA and UK was, and still is, subject to the uncertainty of external factors, notably 'the economics of care'. In the USA she relates how the role of the nurse practitioner was developed by Lorette Ford, a nurse, and Henry Silver, a physician at the University of Colorado with a demonstration project set up in 1965. Stilwell (1996a: 6) suggests that the stimulus for the programme was a shortage of primary health care physicians in the USA in the mid-1960s, which was mirrored in the UK by a similar shortage of general practitioners. Stilwell, drawing on her work with Bowling (Bowling and Stilwell 1988), writes:

> In the UK the response was to improve their [GPs] terms and condi-
> tions of service with a number of measures . . . allowing GPs to claim
> 70% of an employed nurse's salary. GPs were thus encouraged to em-
> ploy practice nurses, and practice nursing was officially recognised as a
> nursing role which could extend primary medical services, through
> assisting doctors.
>
> (Stilwell 1996a: 6)

Shepherd *et al.* (1996), writing from a broadly nursing perspective, comment on arguments which use the fall in general practitioner workforce as an explanation for changes in skill mix in primary care. Drawing on figures cited by Maynard and Bloor (1993), they point out that the 'perceived shortfall' in general practitioner workforce is 'despite rises in the number of GPs from 29,336 in 1980 to 33,839 in 1991' (Shepherd *et al.* 1996: 472), although they acknowledge that 'GPs now undertake . . . diagnostic exami-nations and minor surgical procedures as part of the shift in focus towards primary care' (p. 472). As noted at the outset of the book and in Chapter 1, moves to part-time work and decline in recruitment to training threaten future supply (Carlisle and Johnstone 1996; Taylor and Leese 1997). Gov-ernment policy favours a primary care-led National Health Service and sup-ports a shift in services from secondary to primary care with a corresponding increase in volume of work in general practice, so increasing the need for staff (Pedersen and Leese 1997). A related point is that the transaction costs of operating the recent internal market have not been formally quantified but may be considerable. This is to be distinguished from the moral problem for general practitioners of reconciling personal health care for individuals (the tradition) with health rationing needs arising from the internal market (Royal College of General Practitioners 1996).

However, Shepherd *et al.* (1996) do acknowledge that the development of general practice fundholding created new pressures across broad areas of general practice, for example reductions in secondary care facilities in rural communities. And, certainly, the creation of the National Health Service internal market can, from a medical perspective, be seen as having created difficulties for general practitioners including 'cost containment' (Rashid *et al.* 1996; Lenehan and Watts 1994). It is important to recognize that containment of costs through role substitution does not necessarily mean a cheaper option, as Ridsdale points out (1993: 11). In an experiment (Spitzer *et al.* 1974) carried out by McMasters University, Canada, it was found that nurse practitioners saw half as many patients as family practitioners, and Ridsdale (1993) notes that the model of time allocation described for nurse practitioners by Stilwell (Department of Health 1991a) in the UK seemed to imply a similar ratio of work. Hence the pay differential between nurses and doctors becomes a crucial determinant of cost-effectiveness. Nurses must be paid less than doctors otherwise substitution is not cheaper. However, it is conceivable that nurse practitioners may increase throughput of patients as they become more confident and bring their added value to the service (Mackie 1996; Venning *et al.* 2000), although value beyond meeting targets like throughput is notoriously difficult to measure. Indeed, as one of the NPCRDC study respondents commented: 'The caring component . . . is less measurable. It's very difficult to demonstrate effectiveness . . . and it's actually getting squeezed out.' This point is revisited in Chapter 3.

Cost-effectiveness is, in some respects, a negative term with which to 'sell' role substitution to nursing. One study respondent commented that 'nurses are beginning to feel like commodities which are sold to the highest bidder.' Added to which there are those who take exception to the term 'substitution' and who see nurses as bringing their own nursing dimensions to new work (Anon 1996). As mentioned earlier, the term often used by those who take this position is 'role expansion'. The notion of expansion, as Shepherd *et al.* (1996) comment, has proved attractive to those seeking to rationalize medical tasks in an attempt to contain costs in the secondary care setting. Indeed, the argument that ideas in nursing about expansion of role are expropriated by policy makers to further cost-effectiveness could be equally well made in relation to primary care, so that, as Stilwell (1996a: 6) observes, an obvious conclusion to be drawn is that nursing is shaped in its development by the health system, the role of doctors and the economics of care – an overview of the history of nursing tends to confirm this view.

The literature (research-based papers, policy analyses and commentary) suggests a number of overlapping analyses of the impulse for change in skill mix and role in primary care. Authors highlight at least three areas of analysis: the influence of medicine, ascendancy of nursing arguments, and economic concerns. In each area of analysis, debate reflects a current sense of critical awareness of the uncertain status of professions in respect of both nursing and medicine. Literature sources and study respondents' comments convey a sense of cynicism in relation to cost-cutting and subsequent reconfiguration of role boundaries. Respondents spoke of the insecurity felt by doctors and nurses. One said of medicine, 'it has lost even more than nursing, because its autonomous, untouchable state has now been touched by management'. Louria (1995) commenting from a US perspective writes, 'there are those who argue that the medical profession is going through a traumatic period characterized by loss of autonomy as a consequence of the subversion of doctor–patient relationships'. Bunker (1994) and Hopkins *et al.* (1996), writing from a UK perspective, make a similar point. From a nursing perspective, there are those who are concerned that nurses stand to lose from recent UK health policy changes insofar as they have smaller representation than general practitioners in the recently constituted decision-making primary care groups and their equivalents. Some have claimed that nurses are becoming professionally isolated and need more help if they are going to expand their roles (Cassidy 1996; Hiscock and Pearson 1996). In the words of a study respondent, 'I think what we have now ... is a couple of groups, medicine and nursing ... very dissatisfied, demoralized people who actually don't feel there's much of a future.'

Cynicism is set against a sense of gain and an awareness of the opportunities for nursing, as well as for medicine, as the scene changes in primary care. Running counter to ideas about the uncertainty of professional status are expressions of an awareness of professional contribution, a point explored in some detail in Chapter 5. Expressions of what doctors and nurses stand to lose or gain from boundary changes associated with role substitution can be viewed as reflecting a need to establish and maintain professional identity within an uncertain context. The next chapter takes up this theme, exploring how ideas commonly associated with the 'public good', which historically have characterized professions (Nettleton 1995), are given a distinctive treatment by both nursing and medicine, thus providing some indication of how each profession distinguishes itself in relation to its professional purpose and contribution to primary care.

3 Working on the boundaries: maintaining professional identities in primary care

In this chapter, role substitution (or, as some prefer, role expansion) is examined insofar as it offers the opportunity to explore losses and gains as experienced by doctors and nurses working in primary care. It is through such exploration that we begin to get a sense of how both are establishing professional and other identities within the changing boundaries of primary care. In considering how identities are established it is useful to bear in mind anthropologist Judith Okely's words: 'boundaries may be constructed in unusually elusive ways. Differences can be disguised by similarities and lost in the commonplace' (Okely 1996: 4). When analysing roles and related cultural differences between medicine and nursing in primary care it is tempting to assume differences in identity as simply between the two professions. It is, of course, important to take into account the differences within a profession, as well as between professions. It is also important to take account of ideas, values and beliefs which unite people across professional boundaries as well as within those boundaries: in short to be aware of cultural systems besides those which unite at a professional level.

In order to take account of the complexities of the situation, two case illustrations are offered. In the first, the changing work and role of practice nurses are considered, together with the subsequent impact on community nurses attached to general practices. Uncertainties associated with maintaining and establishing professional identities in a time of change are examined. The increasing identification of practice nurses with preventative work provides a useful focus for the second case illustration in which the impact of government health reforms on general practitioners is explored.

Impact on community nurses of practice nurses' changing roles

Practice nurses have typically been employed by general practitioners, which establishes a particular relationship – one which is different from the relationship between general practitioners and community nurses such as district nurses and health visitors. While district nurses and health visitors may be attached to practices, they are employed by the community trusts. Nevertheless, the employment of practice nurses by general practitioners is not without ambiguities. The term 'employment' is in a sense notional, given that (as noted in Chapter 1) since the GP contract, general practitioners have normally been reimbursed 70 per cent of the salary costs by the health authority. It should also be added that it has been possible for general practitioners to negotiate with their health authority the type of staff they wish to employ and the level of remuneration to be provided.

Marsh and Dawes (1995), in a small but nevertheless key study which investigated the establishment of a 'minor illness nurse' in general practice, write that in England and Wales in 1983 there were 1729 whole-time equivalent practice nurses, rising to 10,157 in 1993 (p.310). General Medical Services statistics show a rise in numbers of practice nurses in England and Wales from 16,743 in 1994 to 19,062 in 1995 (General Medical Services 1995). As indicated in Chapter 2, increase in numbers is attributed to the perceived shortage of general practitioners in the 1960s (Bowling and Stilwell 1988; Stilwell 1996a) and the creation, in the 1990s, by the Conservative administration, of the internal market in primary health care (Ridsdale 1993).

During the 1980s, general practice was heavily focused on quality of care and health promotion. During the 1980s and 1990s, health policy documents (Department of Health and Social Security 1987; Department of Health 1991b, 1992) emphasized the role of disease prevention and health promotion (Nettleton 1995: 229; Quinney and Pearson 1996: 7). The Royal College of General Practitioners (RCGP) produced a series of reports to consider the general practitioner's role in disease prevention and health promotion (Nettleton 1995: 230). Nurses in practices were seen as essential to moving forward on these agendas. The 1990 and 1993 general practice contracts offered specific financial incentives to establish health promotion clinics and programmes which were to be run by practice nurses.

Bowling, writing in the 1996 edition of *The Nurse in Family Practice*, provides useful summaries of the literature, recording how the practice nursing role has evolved since the 1960s. Drawing on the earlier edition of the book (Bowling and Stilwell 1988), she refers to bibliographies of work published between 1967 and 1987, and 1961 and 1987, respectively. She presents an overview of how practice nurses have moved from work centred on the treatment room to work with a preventative focus (Bowling 1996: 15). Cater and Hawthorne (1996) comment that much of the literature, produced between the mid-1960s and mid-1980s, reporting on changes in the practice nurse's role is anecdotal. A review of recent literature mainly con-firms the view that practice nurses have been and are increasingly seen to be identified with preventative work in diverse areas of care which include: giving advice to travellers, child immunization, family planning, registration health checks, well-woman checks, cervical cytology, health checks for people of 75 years and over, well-man checks, management of stress, hypertension, diabetes, asthma, smoking, alcohol and obesity control, and HIV/AIDS advice (Ridsdale 1993; Ross *et al.* 1994; Marsh and Dawes 1995; Paxton *et al.* 1996). In a survey of practice nursing in Glasgow, Peter (1993) comments that health promotion is now considered to be an underlying precept for all practice nursing activities, and while some studies also describe how practice nurses are beginning to undertake minor illness work (Atkin *et al.* 1993; Marsh and Dawes 1995; Rees and Kinnersley 1996), it would appear that prevention of ill health and the promotion of good health are now well established aspects of practice nurses' roles.

Threats to community nurses' professional identity

Some have commented on how the health promotion component of the general practice contract and the consequent increased role for practice nurses in health promotion have been seen by many as a threat for health visitors who see themselves as having a dedicated role in this area of care. Hiscock and Pearson's (1996: 24) research has revealed anxiety amongst community nurses that their responsibilities are being eroded by practice nurses. These authors also note that the community nurses in their study 'expressed great disappointment over the demise of relationships with other community nurses . . . they particularly regretted that these sources of support were disappearing at a time of rapid change and increasing stress' (p. 28).

As the NPCRDC study to explore cultural differences between medicine and nursing in the context of primary care progressed, it became clear that boundary changes were creating uncertainty in relation to professional iden-tity and in connection with aspects of nursing work and role which were seen by the study respondents to be either lost or enhanced. Uncertainty did not appear to be limited straightforwardly to displacement of work between general practitioners and nurses. Rather, we found a knock-on effect creat-ing tensions in communication between different groups of nurses. How-ever, the tensions were not obvious and, in some contrast to fears expressed above, community nurses in the study put forward a positive view of their relationship with practice nurses. One health visitor commented on the reciprocal relationship developing in connection with the immunization of children:

> We don't seem to have any problem with practice nurses . . . Say, with child immunization – they do the jabs in the clinic, we'll do the home

jabs. We'll do jabs in the clinic if necessary and if it's a 'one-off'. There is no conflict. If the practice nurse picks up on something, or if she feels that there's an issue we ought to be involved in (because we probably know the clients better than practice nurses), she will see them [mother and child] as a one-off situation. Then, she [the practice nurse] will keep us informed. For example, she'll say, 'I've seen this lady in the clinic with her child, and there seems to be an issue. Can you contact Mum (to follow up), and is there anything I can be doing if she comes back again?'

In this particular situation, and if the health visitor's words are taken at face value, the community nurses appear to have addressed communication problems and they spoke of having 'very much of an interchange . . . very much of a partnership' with the practice nurses. But this was not always the case. One practice nurse in the study was concerned about the potential for breakdown in communication between practice nurses and community nurses. Resulting complaints from both sides were leading to a situation in which she felt nurses were undermining each other. Other tensions were apparent. The district nurses and health visitors in the study who were attached to general practices were concerned about a loss of professional networking and support. While they felt they had personally gained by a sense of integration with their respective practices, they told us that they knew they were resented by former colleagues in the community.

Relationship between general practice and community health care

Tensions in communication between nurses are not simply that the changing roles of practice nurses impact in a negative way on community nurses. In certain instances this may be the case, but only insofar as practice nurses have been a part of the evolving general practice market culture – a culture which, while it may have been modified by the demise in April 1999 of the National Health Service internal market, cannot easily eradicate its negative legacy. What is critically at stake is the changing relationship between general practice and community health care, a relationship which affects the roles and identities of those involved. And although the comments of the community nurses we interviewed during the course of the study reflect tensions of allegiance to both practice on the one hand and community on the other, the community nurses in our study, both district nurses and health visitors, said, 'We are far more practice orientated as opposed to community orientated'. This statement is not entirely surprising. As Rink *et al.* (1996) point out, citing a paper presented by Morgan at a seminar organized by the National Health Services Management Executive in 1994, 'Recently there have been new initiatives in managing community nursing services within practice boundaries, and in promoting a re-orientation of district nurses and health visitors to the needs of the practice population' (Morgan 1994, cited in Rink *et al.* 1996: 364). What the statement actually meant for the community nurses within our study becomes more explicable when set in the context of their line manager's comments:

> The main thrust of our work is, obviously, to make sure that the GPs have got the right skill mix – district nurses and health visitors doing the right jobs for them. So I see the change. I hate to say it, but I've seen a change in staff loyalties – loyalty first to the GPs and to us second. We deal with the problems. So if the nurses want to be pro-active they don't come to me to say 'is it OK?', which they used to do years ago. They get on and plan it and follow it through with the doctors they are working alongside.

The manager noted that there were problems at the outset of general practice attachment when the district nurses and health visitors were concerned about to whom they were answerable and accountable. She said, 'They've levelled that one out now. They fully understand. Professionally they are accountable to themselves in the first instance, and then they are accountable to the GP and to us [the trust].' She reported that the staff looked to her for professional guidance and leadership which they knew they could not get from the doctors. And, she added, they say they would not like to be employed by the doctors.

It became clear that working in the practices was a source of tension for the community nurses. On the one hand, they spoke of having gained a good teamworking relationship with the general practitioners. They mentioned that they now sat in meetings where their advice was sought. From the community nurses' point of view this indicated an increasing sense of being valued as professionals. On the other hand, it became apparent from talking with the community nurses that the general practitioners were very much in charge of the teams, a point which reflects a more general view (see, for example, Hiscock and Pearson 1996; Long 1996). Indeed, in a group interview it became clear that medical control presented problems for the nurses. One interviewee expressed the opinion that 'the GPs have more to say in what they [practice nurses] do possibly than they do with health visitors and district nurses'. Another member of the group disagreed:

> I think they've got a say in what we do. I think Elspeth [nurse manager] will back me up here. They've even given her a hard time in the past about what staff they want and what they are having . . . and that it's their staff and not Elspeth's staff. Now we're being paid by [the trust], not by the doctors. But they feel that because they are buying our service that they have bought us in if you like, and they can say what we'll do and what we won't do.

She concluded by saying: 'But they let us do our own job . . . and it's more for you [nodding to nurse manager] that the problems have arisen.' It became clear that an underlying concern in this instance was the threat of redundancy. The nurse manager tried to clarify the situation:

From the management point of view it was all about having the right people with the right skills for that practice, and you have to respect that the doctors know what they are talking about. They know their practice population. But it has been a problem for us, because they wanted less . . . If things had gone the wrong way, it could have been a redundancy scenario which, you know, is totally alien to us. But that is the corner we felt we were being pushed into. Mary [community nurse] is right: they [GPs] feel they have now the clout to do that [as fund-holders], which hitherto they haven't.

In relation to the issue of medical control over nursing staff, the nurse manager's words can be read as expressing a concern about potential loss of autonomy and, associated with this, the possibility of losing professional identity 'as health visitors' and 'as district nurses' if general practitioners were to directly employ them. As noted in Chapter 2, the community nurses interviewed felt that being 'attached' to practices rather then being 'employed' offered some protection against being controlled by general practitioners. The district nurse was concerned that the line drawn between her work and the practice nurse's work was being questioned by the general practitioners. Certainly the community nurses we spoke to acknowledged benefits to working together with practice nurses and general practitioners. It became clear that they perceived a common purpose and interest in respect of patients and clients. They enjoyed the sense of teamwork and the potential for improved communication with practice colleagues; and this, as they noted, made a difference to the care their patients and clients received.

The new perceived orientation towards general practice nevertheless presented the community nurses with problems. In trying to analyse why this is the case, it is important to distinguish between the category 'general practitioners' and the category 'general practice'. The latter category goes beyond the personalities involved. The community nurses' concerns about potential redundancy and associated concerns about overlap between their work and the work of practice nurses exemplify Hiscock and Pearson's (1996) point (cited in Chapter 2) that fundholding did not fit comfortably into the purchaser/provider distinction. The authors suggest that there is tension in situations where general practitioners working 'as colleagues' in primary health care teams encounter primary care and community health care nurses who they may have directly employed or whose services they purchased (Hiscock and Pearson 1996: 24).

In the relationship between general practice and community health care, professional identity appears to matter. The community nurses felt their professional identity to be under threat not because there is a lack of willingness on the part of nurses to work with general practitioners or because the latter are unwilling to recognize nurses' skills and knowledge. The problem lies with the structure of the relationship between general practice and community care. In a research-based paper, Traynor (1995) highlights the uncertainty and declining morale and job satisfaction amongst community nurses, and contrasts this with the relative job satisfaction of practice nurses. In part, this appears to be as a consequence of the uncertainty and associated lack of infrastructure for community care identified by Singh *et al.* (1996). Uncertainty in relation to professional identity also appears to be a consequence of the once strongly evolving internal market within general practice and the changing relationship between general practice and community care which affects the identities of those involved. One reading of both the literature and respondents' comments is that they are expressions of a tension between allegiance to profession on the one hand and allegiance to place of work on the other.

Uncertainty in relation to professional identity: the broad picture

We found that nurses reflect on the tension between allegiance to profession and allegiance to place of work. The literature (both research-based and commentary) and our respondents' observations suggest that nurses are aware of the need for a review of inflexible roles and work boundaries based too strongly on professional interest. As one senior nurse respondent observed, 'there has had to be a concerted attack on the professions because the only way in which general management could deliver the agenda was to dismantle the power of doctors and nurses in the hospital.' It is generally accepted that the Griffiths Report (Department of Health and Social Security 1983) introduced the role of general management into the National Health Service. Cox (1991) writes that the 'pressures to bring management to the top of the National Health Service agenda had been building up steadily throughout the 1970s' (p. 93). He observes that many commentators saw the desire to obtain some managerial control over doctors as being a principal objective of the changes heralded by the Griffiths Report, although, as Cox writing in 1991 suggests, there is doubt that general management initiatives instigated by Griffiths substantially affected the behaviour of doctors. Indeed, Scrivens's (1988) work has shown how general managers have involved medical staff in policy and resource discussions, appointing clinical directors and heads of specialities to be accountable in this respect to a unit general manager. The 1989 White Paper (Department of Health 1989) proposals for self-governing, revenue-earning clinicians within primary and acute care together with the constitution of an internal market provided a climate within which doctors could become entrepreneurs. Recent White Papers (for example, Department of Health 1998; Welsh Office 1998a) provide, perhaps, the strongest management challenge to doctors, although their actual impact on diminishing the power and status of doctors remains to be seen.

In contrast, general management has had a 'traumatic effect . . . on the management of nurses and the roles of most senior nurses' (Cox 1991: 101). Robinson (1992) notes that the introduction of general management through Griffiths resulted in senior nurses at district and regional levels of the health service losing their jobs. Thus control over the nursing budget was lost and line management control of nursing was lost. Walby *et al.*, commenting on Robinson's contribution to an analysis of the effects of general management on nursing, write:

> Robinson addresses the lack of interest in nursing policy issues, and this despite the size of the workforce – half a million. This lack of interest she labels 'the black hole theory of nursing'. While the Griffiths reforms were certainly intended to control medicine, nursing was merely 'caught in the cross fire'.
>
> (1994: 143–4)

Nurses are aware of the attack on professions, and there is concern that the attack continues to disproportionately disadvantage nursing. For example, a recent proposal for a future health care workforce draws on ideas about designing care on the basis of patient need rather than on the basis of existing role demarcations (Health Services Management Unit 1996). The notion of a flexible generic worker is elaborated in response to the following question: If we were designing the workforce today for tomorrow's health service, what would it look like? (Health Services Management Unit 1996: 19). In relation to primary care, the proposal suggests that a broadly based generic workforce should be designed from a review of the workload currently undertaken by the wide range of staff working within primary health care – for example nurse practitioners, health visitors, district nurses and midwives.

It is claimed that the proposal will foster flattened structures and a non-hierarchical approach to health care. However, there are at least two major problems with the proposal in relation to primary health care. First, the flattening of hierarchical relationships depends on where you are standing. The general practitioner is given prominence in the proposal. Statements about putting patient needs and the demands of a service above traditional role demarcations do not extend to medical practitioners. Certainly from a nursing perspective, old hierarchies are reinforced rather than flattened. The second problem is this: while inflexible professional boundaries may impede the provision of care based on patient need, there is a danger that a breakdown in professional boundaries might actually be counterproductive. As indicated earlier, Hiscock and Pearson (1996) elaborate this danger, emphasizing how lack of professional networking can lead to demoralization and a sense of diminished autonomy. Respondents' concerns that 'things have gone too far' imply that a diminution of professional identity and autonomy can be dysfunctional in identifying a particular 'professional' contribution to meet patient need and service demand in primary health care. A similar point has been made about medicine in relation to the changing boundaries of care (Hopkins *et al.* 1996).

Thus what is an advantage from one perspective (i.e. the breakdown of inflexible professional boundaries) is, from another perspective, seen as creating uncertainty, vulnerability and a sense of isolation and increasing stress (Cassidy 1996a; Hiscock and Pearson 1996). This, in turn, may lead to unproductive behaviour such as breakdown in communication between colleagues which, as one of our nurse commentators suggested, leads nurses to undermine each other. The latter respondent was referring to the relationship between community nurses and practice nurses which, as stated earlier, has been recognized in the literature as an area of tension (Wiles and Robinson 1994; Gibbings 1995; Ross *et al.* 1995).

The purpose of the case illustration was to discuss how role change in one category of nurses creates tensions that ripple throughout the profession. Discussion has moved from the everyday experiences of nurses who are touched by change through to recognition of wider issues relating to the broad context within which nurses practise. The issue of the current attack on professions is critical in this respect. In recent years, nurses and doctors have confronted the challenge to their perceived professional power and influence from National Health Service general management. As discussed, nurses have fared worse than doctors in moves to control professionals within the health service. For nurses, the attack on their professional status is intimately tied to the logistics of the provision of health care. As Davies (1995) has noted: 'staffing the service takes precedence over educating the nurse' (p. 126). Frank Dobson's comments on nurse education is a case in point. Early in 1999, Mr Dobson (then Secretary of State for Health) publicly stated his concern that nurse education ill prepares nurses for their future work. He was also concerned that the entry criteria might deny many who would like to care for people the opportunity to do so. There is a suggestion in these comments that nursing in higher education is élitist and thus nurse education might be better placed outside the higher education sector. It is worth noting here that to take nurse education out of higher education may actually undermine one of the greatest democratizing processes ever to influence UK higher education. The entry of nursing education en masse over recent years into universities has increased the number of entrants with non-traditional qualifications and it has increased the number of women in higher education at all levels.

This aside, the counterarguments to the Secretary of State's point of view are obvious. Many have been rehearsed and some published (for example, Butterworth 1999; Howard 1999; Martin 1999; Rafferty 1999). Important amongst these is recognition that caring and compassion require competence. The public will be best served by a competent, confident and well educated nursing workforce – nurses who understand the policy issues and who are prepared and able to engage with other health care professionals in providing high quality, evidence-based patient care. As suggested, there are a number of factors which make the realization of these aspirations an up-hill struggle and which could impact negatively on patient care, not least the erosion of a sense of professional identity.

Government reforms and general practitioners

The increasing identification of practice nurses with preventative work provides a useful focus for considering the impact of government reforms on general practitioners. From one perspective, general practitioners can be viewed as active agents in the changing role of practice nurses insofar as they delegate and supervise the work of practice nurses. From another perspective, general practitioners, themselves, can be viewed as the some-what passive participants in a process of policy-driven changes to reverse the orthodox 'professional order', a process which modifies ideas about service and the public good with the ideals of enterprise culture; replacing the passive patient with the active consumer of health, and replacing profes-sional divisions with integrated structures for the delivery of health care (Keat 1991; Fournier 1997).

Much of the preventative work delegated to practice nurses has a 'family' focus, including family planning, women's health, child health, assessments of older people, advice about lifestyle and health promotion. Family medi-cine has featured as an aspect of prevention in general practice at least since the inception of the National Health Service (Davies 1984), when, in effect, general practice appealed to the idea of prevention in order to establish its professional identity at a time when the emphasis was on curing (Armstrong 1979; Nettleton 1995). As discussed in Chapter 1, general practitioners strove to distinguish their work from that of the hospital doctors whose emphasis was on curing and technological intervention. General practice was seen as having an inadequate research base and its practitioners looked for a distinct body of knowledge on which they could base their expertise. Explanations of the growth in family medicine and the emphasis on prevention in rela-tion to general practice include the view that general practitioners have utilized those ideas in order to find a distinctive identity within medicine. Sociologists have also observed how medicine, including general practice medicine, has sought to increase its constituency and its surveillance of that constituency through a process commonly referred to as the medicalization of everyday life (see Foucault 1973, 1977, 1980; Illich 1975; Bloor and McIntosh 1990; Armstrong 1995). The medicalization of everyday life can also be seen as part of what Fournier (1997), drawing on Abbott (1988), refers to as the 'cultural work' the professions engage in to protect their jurisdiction. Fournier notes how 'Abbott uses this notion of "cultural work" to refer to the strategies that professions deploy to manipulate their systems of knowledge in such a way that they can appropriate various problems as falling under their juris-diction' (Fournier 1997: 7).

A complicating component of explanations of the growth of family medi-cine or the medicine of everyday life problems which, in turn, increases pressure on general practice work is the idea that people no longer rely on doctors for health information which is now readily available through vari-ous media. We have already noted that some would argue that the author-ity of doctors, together with scientists, is challenged (Beck 1992; Williams and Calnan 1996). However, this does not necessarily mean that patients do not consult general practitioners. Rather it may be the case that, far from curtailing the doctor's sphere of work and influence, media interest in-creases medical influence as the public become more alerted to medical problems. Taking the idea of 'sovereign consumer' (Keat and Abercrombie 1991) to its logical conclusion, it might mean that patients increasingly see the general practitioner's advice as an option (cf. Gabe and Calnan 1989) rather than a prescription in what may become a process of shopping around for medical information and services.

Thus, at one and the same time, family medicine is increasing and, some would argue, diminishing in importance. Insofar as it is increasing and nurses are delegated family or preventative work, it could be argued that we see a blurring of boundaries and the possibility of interdisciplinary teamworking. However, insofar as the area of work passing to practice nurses is, perhaps, losing its importance then another reading emerges. And, as with the de-cline in importance of temperature recording with the advent of antibiotics, it could be argued that 'family work' is being passed on to nurses. From a medical perspective, this could be seen as a perfectly appropriate develop-ment for practice nurses, as well as a gain for general practitioners insofar as it potentially allows for the development of other aspects of general practice work. Marsh and Dawes's (1995) words regarding the training of practice nurses are interesting in this respect: 'Nursing and midwifery training and practice, *plus experience as a mother* provided satisfactory basic knowledge for the nurse' (p. 779, emphasis added). It has been suggested that medicine has been increasingly extending its province to conditions that would have been dealt with thirty years ago through family networks (Fox 1993; Nettleton 1995), however the suggestion that general practitioners' experiences as mothers might provide part of their required knowledge base does not, to the best of my knowledge, appear in the literature.

The suggestion that experience as a mother might provide satisfactory basic knowledge for the nurse is from one perspective quite sensible. Ex-perience is important and a mother's experience is no doubt to be taken seriously. However, the words cited sit uneasily with ideas about profes-sional contribution and, since they are directed at practice nurses and not at general practice as a whole, they exemplify Davies's (1995) point that we live in a society divided by sex which defines nursing as women's work. Following Davies, while the words 'experience as a mother' do not necessarily devalue individual nurses, they do devalue nursing and are an expression of the patriarchy that informs how the relationship between doctors and nurses has been and still is being constructed.

Enterprise culture and the holistic ideal

It is not simply that the delegation of family work (now seen as less of a challenge to medicine) is a manifestation of the power of doctors *vis-à-vis* nurses and an expression of incipient patriarchy; rather, the delegation of family work may be a reflection of how a profession challenged by the climate of enterprise, a legacy of the 1989 White Paper, has tried to establish itself as a profession whose extended domain is the market. With the internal market, general practitioners were well placed to utilize nurses to a practice's advantage. Indeed Roland's (1996) editorial is an expression of how a profession was only very recently thinking about its future in terms of enterprise culture. Roland points out that if general practitioners were to insist that boundaries should be drawn around their responsibilities and that they 'contract separately for services outside a defined core' of responsibilities, then they would face competition from providers as diverse as acute trusts, community trusts, ambulance trusts – all of whom would presumably employ general practitioners to do much of the work'. Roland continues, 'General practitioners, who, as fundholders, have grown used to using the internal market would find the full force of the market turned on them' (1996: 704).

Thus the shift in work from doctor to nurse can be analysed in different ways depending on one's viewpoint. From a market perspective, it makes sense for doctors to use nurses to a practice's full advantage. From a perspective which looks critically at issues of sex as they bear on the relationship between doctors and nurses, there are inequities in the process.

There is also, however, a sense in which general practitioners experience a loss as work moves to practice nurses. Indeed, the loss is expressed not merely in terms of personal loss, but also in what general practitioners sense as a loss to patients. One general practitioner we interviewed commented that 'disease is about dealing with families'. From her point of view, nurses who took over health promotion and prevention in special areas were 'cutting into a GP's relationship with the holistic care of a family'. She explained:

> Our work is defined by relationships . . . and if you say [referring to a patient] well actually she's got this disease, she should go to that clinic [run by practice nurse]. Then that cuts across our whole approach which is about relationships and people and its about working with disease . . .
> If the practice nurse is, say, dealing with all the asthma then she is not seeing the whole – the mother, perhaps going through a divorce or

an affair or something that might affect the asthma. Equally, you don't have an opportunity as a GP to see the mother alongside the child when she is apparently well. So you are losing opportunities.

These words, which broadly accord with contributors to the literature including Richardson and Maynard (1995), and Garbett (1996a), are interesting in that they link ideas about disease and pathology with family events and processes. They also suggest a connection between those ideas and other ideas about taking into account the whole situation and, importantly, connect an understanding of disease to an understanding of relationships. The words also convey a hint of concern for the potential loss to patients should a holistic 'generalist' perspective be compromised by work undertaken by nurses who provide 'specialist' care such as given in, for example, asthma clinics as cited above.

Of course, nurses use the word holistic to describe the care they give (May 1991, 1992). When pressed to distinguish how her care might differ from the care given by a doctor, a practice nurse who was interviewed for our study suggested:

I think they do deal with caring. I think the whole holistic approach of medicine is caring, but I feel they care more from a treatment point of view. They care enough to listen to the symptoms and they get them [patients] the best possible treatment . . . The nursing care comes more from the emotional side.

There are different types of care. And their [the doctors] care is in getting the treatment, the diagnosis . . . where nursing care is more from the social point of view and more on a level as well. I do think lots of patients see doctors as being up on a pedestal whereas the patients tell me 'I can talk to you because you're more like us'.

In some respects, the nurse's words echo May's (1991, 1992) findings from interviews with staff nurses working with terminally ill patients. May noted that the nurses accounted for the care they gave in terms of knowing the patients and knowing them as individuals or whole persons (May 1992: 473). Fagermoen (1997) writes:

Realising the value of being a fellow human may be a precondition for reciprocal trust, as this was identified in interactions characterised by mutual sharing of personal experiences. The value of integrity was reflected in actions emphasising the patient as a whole being with a past, present and future.

(p. 239)

The idea of relationship is important here. Connections between care and relationships were implicit in the responses of other respondents. For example, one general practitioner, reflecting on changes between medicine and midwifery, spoke of regret in 'losing midwifery cases'. He emphasized how the partners in the practice 'used to handle midwifery cases because they liked the relationships'. He added that, 'there was never any evidence that doctors did it better than midwives . . . it was probably the other way round'. Continuing, he noted in regretful tone, 'In this practice, now, we've let it go and . . . well, in a way I feel I've lost it.' His comments on how patients might feel about the change are interesting:

> Some have strong loyalties, others wouldn't care very much. It's like everything else, people are different, and so what is someone's loss is someone else's gain. But on the whole I suspect we will recover new relationships, and new things will be done by all of us. I mean, it's like a sort of, I think there's a care control revolution taking place. So I think the future's for nurses.

However, this particular general practitioner expressed concern that nurses might be impeding development of their holistic perspective (a point raised earlier in connection with nurses as potential partners in general practice), a perspective held by Salvage (1995). He was referring to district nurses, but his concern was for the wider issue of maintaining a generalist approach in the face of the increase of specialist services, as the following commentary indicates:

> General practitioners see themselves first . . . as a person who makes an initial decision. Whereas nurses very often are saying 'that's not for me, that's for the psychiatric nurse . . . that's for the stoma nurse, or the diabetic nurse', and I just find myself wondering if they are pursuing that too far . . . Are they impeding their development as a holistic visitor?

One reading of the foregoing discussion is that both doctors and nurses are concerned with relationships, and with taking a holistic perspective on the care they give. In common with each other, there is appeal to ideas about the worth of others. Overall, the words convey a belief in the virtue of pursuing the public good – a sense of the altruism historically attributed to the professional role (Nettleton 1995).

There are differences, however, between the meanings attributed by doctors and nurses to the connections to be made between holism, relationship and care. Doctors apply ideas about disease and pathology to ideas about holism, relationship and caring, whereas nurses apply ideas about knowing the person and mutual sharing of experiences. The words of the first general practitioner cited above suggest that holism has to do with the whole situation, whereas nursing the whole person is a fairly common expression in nursing literature pertaining to nurse/patient relationships (Spooner 1995; Fagermoen 1997).

It could be said that if general practitioners are holistic in terms of dealing with the overall 'medical' status of patients, then they need to be generalist in their skills. If nurses are holistic in terms of dealing with patients' emotional and social needs it could be argued that they do not need to be generalist, but that they can take account of emotional and social needs in relation to particular conditions or diseases. In short, they act as specialists in relation to the condition. It is interesting to note that very little discussion of holism in connection with generalism appears in the literature, whereas links are made between holism and specialism: for example, the psychiatric clinical specialist in the home care setting (Ward-Miller 1996), the specialist nurse in HIV/AIDS medicine (Whitehead 1996), the specialist status of orthopaedic nursing (Love 1995) and holistic care in relation to the menopause (Choi 1995).

However, even the distinction (between nursing and medicine) in meanings attributed to the idea of holism does not hold unconditionally. There is some evidence in the literature of an interest, by general practitioners, in the whole patient (Heath 1995), particularly in the international literature (Ashby *et al*. 1996; Hurst 1996; Kocurek 1996). In relation to the idea of role substitution, it is useful to note that training for new roles in nursing may encourage a reconceptualization of clinician/client relationships. Also, while it is possible to identify broad differences between medicine and nursing in the interpretation and treatment of core values, differences may be less easy to discern where doctors and nurses occupy the same space, as for example, in teams and teamworking (Gillman *et al*. 1996). To take another example: earlier discussion touched on how some community nurses felt a growing sense of affiliation to the general practices to which they were attached rather than to the trusts which employed them. To reiterate what the nurse manager said, 'I hate to say it, but I've seen a change in staff loyalties – first to the GPs and to us second'.

Culture clash?

The expressions of loss recorded in this chapter suggest a sense of regret that both doctors and nurses cannot make more of holism as well as other hard-to-define aspects of care. As one of our respondents pointed out, 'despite the fact that nurses are trained in holism, the concept is totally unmarketable in the current climate'. A similar sentiment is expressed by Salvage (1995), who has suggested that some of the values of nursing, such as compassion and social justice, are no longer possible. Garbett (1996b) states that nursing is losing the heart of what it once did. One possible explanation for this is the increasing tendency to value what is measurable rather than to measure what is valuable. It is certainly easier in the current climate of health service provision to value what can be demonstrated quantitatively in performance indicators as effective, both clinically and in terms of cost, rather than to measure hard-to-define relational aspects of care such as compassion. However, this is not to say that compassion will not be measured, packaged and marketed in the future. An article in the *Times Higher Educational Supplement* reported that medical students at Brown University, USA, will now have to prove they have compassion in addition to a command of scientific facts (Marcus 1997: 9). The demand for proof of compassion comes from the public – an instance, perhaps, of how the interests of the articulate consumer can help to shape professional agendas.

Discussion within this chapter has drawn attention to ways in which values, ideas and beliefs broadly conceived as the culture of profession (bearing in mind, however, that the culture of profession is not exclusively one of commitment to the public good, as noted in the following chapter) are juxtaposed with values, ideas and beliefs associated with enterprise in the changing climate of primary care. We might wish to speculate that general practitioners are in a stronger position than nurses to manage the sometimes conflicting ideas insofar as they have had experience of being both purchasers and providers of health care, and also by virtue of their 'special' status in primary care. They continue to be named as the leaders in a primary care-led National Health Service. As noted in Chapter 1, this could change, hence we sense uncertainty on the part of some doctors as well as nurses. As one general practitioner told us: 'I think possibly the nurse's role is developing even more quickly than the general practitioner's, although I don't think they've found it yet – any more than we have.' He was referring in this instance to nursing's role in primary care, a role which appears to be elusive to some nurses. One interviewee, a nurse, said:

What have they [nurses] gained? Maybe a few salary rises. They are in the news a lot. They get media coverage, and they will always have the respect of the public. I think they are in a state of transition and confusion. I don't see one gain. I don't personally see that nursing or nurses have gained anything within the primary care situation, other than a sea of confusion.

The tension between, on the one hand, ideas associated with professional duty and purpose and, on the other hand, ideas associated with enterprise culture makes for vulnerability and uncertainty, creating a cultural milieu which I term 'boundary culture' and which is explored further in Chapter 4.

4 Boundary culture: exploring a realm of uncertainty

Anthropologists have long theorized about the innovative and creative possibilities of ambiguous spaces or, as Turner (1977) describes them, 'betwixt and between positions assigned by law, custom, convention and ceremonial' (p. 95). It is possible to speculate that health care reforms have created such ambiguous spaces. Both general practitioners and nurses have expressed excitement at the possibilities emerging in primary health care, and there is evidence to suggest creativity and innovation. For example, innovations in primary health care nursing are listed in Ross and Elliott's (1995) excellent review and update (Elliott 1998) and include models for developing user-focused services, health of the nation targets, care management and assessment strategies, as well as joint initiative responses to care challenges such as the management of chronic disease. Innovation in the form of nurse practitioner projects is now common, and there are a number of examples within the UK and beyond including those reported by Dowling *et al.* (1995), Ruiz *et al.* (1995), Dontje *et al.* (1996), Lewis (1996) and Reveley (1998). The opportunities for exploiting the potential for innovation are discussed fully in Chapter 5. However, as indicated in earlier chapters, despite expressions of a sense of liberation (Denner 1995; Healy 1996) and opportunity (Bowling and Stilwell 1996; Garbett 1996b), there exists for general practitioners and more especially for nurses an overwhelming sense of loss and uncertainty. It is this finding, specifically insofar as it relates to primary care nursing, that provides the focus for this chapter.

The problem of uncertainty has been described as 'inherent to medicine in general' (Fox and Swazey 1974). Uncertainty in this respect has been discussed, for example, in relation to therapeutic interventions like transplantation. A classic and sensitive sociological exposition on the subject of uncertainty in relation to transplantation is Renée Fox's (1974) book *Experiment Perilous* in which she observes the stresses not only for the physicians in her study but also for the patients who faced such uncertain outcomes. Fox describes how both came to terms with the uncertainties they faced.

Themes common to both the physicians' and patients' mechanisms for coming to terms included group support, not only within but also between physician and patient groups. Indeed, patients were known by physicians as patient-colleagues (Fox 1974: 89). Another important theme to emerge from Fox's research with Swazey (1974) was 'the courage to fail', by which is implied the courage it takes for patients to face uncertain outcomes and the courage it takes for physicians to recognize they may fail to heal – especially those physicians who are working on the outer boundaries of what is known and pushing beyond them (Fox and Swazey 1974: 318). Both themes are relevant to a discussion of how to deal with uncertainty and as such are revisited in the section 'Training for uncertainty' in Chapter 5.

Of interest to discussion in this present chapter is what appears to be a lack of exploration of the basis of uncertainty within primary care generally and primary care nursing in particular. The uncertain status of the future for health care and nursing is recognized in, for example, the report *Healthcare Futures* (Warner *et al.* 1998) commissioned by the United Kingdom Central Council for Nursing, Midwifery and Health Visiting (UKCC). As will become evident below, there has also been work which explores uncertainties faced by nurses in acute care settings. There are a number of overlapping factors which contribute to uncertainty and which may impair the potential for innovation in primary care nursing. Important amongst these are the problems associated with maintaining professional identity as discussed in Chapter 3. In this present chapter, two further factors are discussed. They are first, the difficulties associated with working in a risk environment, especially uncertainty in relation to the changing status of patients and clients. This is a factor which, as has been hinted in the preceding chapters, is taking on increasing importance in discussions about health care provision. The second factor addressed is uncertainty in relation to the operation of new nursing roles, including training and leadership strategies for new roles. As is the case in previous chapters, discussion of these two key factors draws on the literature review and empirical research undertaken in the study described in the Introduction. It is followed by a review of the ideas which appear to underpin uncertainty in respect of primary care nursing, and which, together with our other findings, assist an understanding of ideas and values which impact on the changing boundary between medicine and nursing.

Working in a risk environment: uncertainty in relation to patients

A contributing factor to nurses' uncertainty is explored by Annandale (1996), who writes that nurses may feel insecure about how their work and responsibilities relate not only to those of other professionals, but also to the rights and expectations of patients. Bolman (1995) makes a similar point in relation to doctors in the USA. Annandale's discussion is based on a study of the legal accountability of nurses and midwives. The research was undertaken in late 1994 in secondary care settings, where tasks such as drug administration and, more recently, venipuncture, cannulation and the administration of intravenous drugs are seen as producing insecurity insofar as patients, increasingly aware of their rights, are viewed as a potential source of risk (Annandale 1996: 422).

From one perspective, that patients are aware of their rights would appear to be a positive development, and the nurses in Annandale's account acknowledged this. However, the author reports how a 'sense that patients and relatives are "looking over the nurse's shoulders" undoubtedly generates personal vigilance over the nurse's or midwife's actions and the actions of others' (Annandale 1996: 423). Annandale interprets this kind of felt surveillance as a reflection of nurses' insecurity about their competence in relation to new tasks and roles, and comments on how this may be understood as a function in the shift in relations from producer to consumer that contemporary social theorists have suggested is characteristic of late modern society (for example, she cites Abercrombie 1994).

Annandale (1996) suggests that nurses and midwives may overestimate the true risk of experiencing a complaint or malpractice suit, as the statistics reveal that they are not very common given the immense nursing workforce. However, she makes the point that felt experience of risk has its consequences, and one consequence is that while nurses write about creating partnerships with patients and clients, the reality is that partnerships are hard to foster when patients and clients are simultaneously seen as risk generators. The paper provides a useful critique of assumptions about the ease with which nurses establish relationships with clients, and provides a salutary reminder that uncertainty and insecurity affect working relationships.

While concerns about patient surveillance were not expressed overtly by the NPCRDC study respondents, concerns were expressed obliquely in comments by nurses such as, 'when nurses do move forward and develop their roles, they do so on a very insubstantial basis'. An example of how this might be the case was offered by a nurse respondent who said, 'I do worry about pharmacology. What is the pharmacology base of nursing? Many of these practice nurses did the old SRN with 26 weeks of theoretical background, science, whatever you want to call it, of which precious little was pharmacology based.' The consumer respondent's comments are apposite here. The following point was made, and reiterated throughout the interview, in relation to the questions posed about areas of work moving from doctors to nurses in primary care: 'I think what the nursing profession has to get to grips with is that the public don't necessarily worry about who does the task, what they want is the task done by a competent person, and that's the key issue.'

In relation to the latter point, there is a substantial body of literature which suggests that patients want continuity of care with a specific professional

(Freeman and Richards 1993; Sweeney and Gray 1995). There is also evidence to suggest that some women prefer a woman clinician (Brooks and Phillips 1996). However, the point made usefully draws attention to patient or consumer confidence in changing roles. Concern about consumer confidence in relation to changing roles was expressed by a study respondent, a general practitioner, who stressed that nurses might not have the education and experience to spot problems which, while covert and not stressed by patients, could be important (see also Richardson and Maynard 1995; Garbett 1996a). Nurses are also concerned about lack of education for new roles, as indicated in the following interview extract:

> Nurses themselves are often quite frightened of these extended roles. I think there is a crisis situation which nurse education has to face. I think nurse education is failing the profession at the moment. I think they have got to get their act together. They are not producing learning that the service needs, and they are certainly not producing somebody that feels tremendously confident in relation to their actual competences with patients. They [students] might be good at writing things; they might be good at passing certain exams, but when I speak to them [nurses] they sit there and say, 'I really sometimes wonder whether I should be doing this. I'm not competent you know. I sometimes ask the question, what if it went wrong, you know? Would I really be able to stand up in a court of law and say I was confident I had all the preparation I needed to do that?'

Here, implicit reference is being made to the United Kingdom Central Council Code of Professional Conduct which requires nurses to be accountable for their actions and only to participate in care for which they are prepared, competent and confident to administer (UKCC 1992a). If nurses do not think they are prepared, competent and confident to administer a particular type of care, then from the UKCC's perspective they are correct in refusing to participate. However, they also risk the accusation of being unwilling to take on responsibility. As one general practitioner in the study said:

> When the chips are down, the nurse retreats to saying 'I am a nurse and you're the doctor'. And no matter how senior they [nurses] are, when things start to go wrong, what they say is 'this is as far as I can go, and now I have to hand over to a doctor'. For example, we have an experienced midwife who hands over to an inexperienced doctor, and that seems most odd, most odd.

The example cited may not be representative, and certainly it is an example which does not hold true for all nurses and midwives in all situations. Nevertheless, it is a further reflection of the uncertainties that exist both within and outside the nursing profession about emerging innovative roles (see Cowley 1995; Hall *et al.* 1995; Smith-Regojo 1995, for further illustrations).

Uncertainty in relation to new roles

Rashid *et al.* (1996) point out that there appears to be considerable confusion among general practitioners, nurses and National Health Service managers about when to use the term practice nurse and when to use the term nurse practitioner. They stress that whereas within the context of general practice, a practice nurse implements prescribed programmes of care, working under the supervision of a general practitioner, a nurse practitioner is usually qualified to degree level and works autonomously alongside a general practitioner colleague. This definition accords in part with Bowles's (1992) description of a nurse practitioner as a nurse working alongside general practitioners (with them, not for them) as an autonomous provider of health care in the setting of general practice. Kaufmann's (1996: 44) definition, drawing, as he acknowledges, on the work of Pickersgill (1995), adds that as well as being independent and autonomous, nurse practitioners are educated to an 'advanced level'.

However, this last point concerning level of education is contentious. This is reflected in recent commentary on the release of the United Kingdom Central Council's interim paper on the nature of advanced practice (Healy 1996; Mathieson 1996). Mathieson reports on the response of nurse practitioners to the paper which was read at the fourth international nurse practitioner conference. The paper suggests that 'advanced practitioners should be small in number, renamed "nurse consultants" and prepared to masters or doctorate level. They would be assessed by a panel of peers, in the same way as the medical royal colleges assess senior doctors.' The paper goes on to suggest that nurse practitioners are doctor substitutes who carry out an inadequately researched and poorly understood role. Their work and role according to the paper, as Mathieson reports it, does not represent advanced practice, and only in some cases approximates to specialist practice (Mathieson 1996: 15).

Nurse practitioners' responses have been of anger and frustration at the paper's failure to accept them as advanced, or even specialist, practitioners. Healy (1996) reporting on a conference on the issue of advanced practice held in October 1996 by the United Kingdom Central Council, states that the conference was told that 'debates around advanced practice always came back to the role of nurse practitioners'. Most people felt that nurse practitioners had yet to be formally acknowledged. The general view was that most operated at a specialist rather than an advanced level. Whether specialist or advanced practitioners, there is confusion about the role. One nurse respondent in the NPCRDC study reported that she knew 'about sixty different titles that nurses were using in relation to advanced practice'. She continued:

> So if you think they're confused, think about the patients and the doctors. You know, if you said to a trust chief exec., 'do you realize that

you have twenty people in your organization that are using this title?'
they wouldn't have a clue what they [the titles] meant or what they
[the nurses] did . . . And neither would nursing. So there's a real danger
of confusion unless someone does something.

There are a number of readings to be made of this aspect of the written
commentary on nurse practitioners. One reading is that at the heart of the
controversy lies the matter of status within the profession, and associated
with this the vexed issue of what constitutes a nurse or what is nursing.
These questions were first alluded to by Florence Nightingale and they continue to be posed by contemporary nurses, including our respondents for
this study. The nurse practitioner role has, as Stilwell (1996a) and others
(for example, Ridsdale 1993) point out, been associated with physician shortage in the USA and Canada. This in turn has led to a call for more nurse
practitioners (Ditzenberger *et al.* 1995; Hoffman and Redman 1995). Within
the UK, talk of the nurse practitioner role as an extension of the practice nurse
role and its consequent medical influence has resulted in some deprecation
of those who could be seen to be aspiring to be junior doctors. Indeed, as
Stilwell points out this was the case in the USA in the 1960s. She writes:

> Given that a physician shortage was the impetus for the development of
> the nurse practitioner role in the US, it is not altogether surprising that
> the nurse practitioners were perceived by many nurses there as aspiring
> to be junior doctors. Indeed these early nurse practitioners were acting
> as substitutes for family physicians. (Stilwell 1996a: 7)

Stilwell continues, drawing on Deveraux (1991), 'defendants of the role
asserted that nurse practitioners were a reflection of the nursing profession's
increasing concern throughout the 1960s with improving clinical nursing
practice and meeting the needs of people with no access to health care'
(Stilwell 1996a: 7).

It is interesting to note how Hancock, writing in 1997, defends the role in
the UK in a similar manner. She suggests that in the UK, 'nurse practitioners
could contract to deliver a wide range of services for homeless people living
on the streets who are not registered with a GP' (Hancock 1997: 17). Similarly, a senior nurse respondent in the present study made reference to how
nurses might initiate a 'proper primary health care'. Commenting on the
present system she said, 'it's all about medically oriented health care, and it
isn't proper primary health care – it's not World Health Organization primary health care. It's basically delivering medical services in a community
rather than in an institutional setting.'

Another respondent commented similarly on the potential for nurse
practitioners as primary care practitioners, nurses 'who are proactive in relation to the needs of a population', for example a practice population. She
observed how 'a lot of primary care nurses . . . have lost their understanding
of primary prevention', and she continued:

I think the way that the service has gone has been very much one of reacting to what comes through the door, delivering . . . care, delivering packages of care, packages of care for this and that, for example diabetes. And its striking how many [nurses] you talk to don't understand the basis of immunization. They know it goes on, but if you actually press them on what it's doing, and what it's supposed to do . . . and about all the things around epidemiology . . . there isn't, really, an understanding of that public health role which is really a health-driven system. And, to me, it's about not just tasks; it's about strengthening that knowledge and understanding to a level where what you produce is a thinking, autonomous practitioner who isn't just reacting to what comes through the door, but is actually being very proactive in looking at the needs of a population, and saying, 'if I'm working in the inner city, then there are certain things this practice must be doing because otherwise no wonder we are being overwhelmed by this problem because we are doing absolutely nothing.'

The sentiment expressed in these words is reflected in various writings (Ashton and Seymour 1988; Department of Health 1993a, b; Neufer 1994), but perhaps more directly by Peckham and Winters (1996) who put forward the idea that community health nurses in the UK feel that their public health role is marginalized by general practice-centred primary care rather than community-based primary care. There is a sense in which primary care conceived of as public health is viewed as something nursing has lost, but it is seen as a dimension of care that nurses might usefully pursue, as discussed in Chapter 5.

Hancock (1997) and others defend the nurse practitioner as unequivocally a nursing role. However, uncertainty about nursing and new nursing roles was expressed by our nursing respondents in one form or another, for example: 'I'm not sure what the nursing profession is trying to do', and 'I'm not sure where nursing is going, and there are calls for advanced skills and advanced practice . . . I'm not sure that I know what that means.' Concern was also voiced about how far responsibility actually follows new work and roles and the role of the United Kingdom Central Council in regulating practice and accountability for practice:

The actual body [UKCC] that regulates the profession has not articulated what they think these changing roles should be, or what sort of training they need to perform them. What signifies advanced practice, they have not really outlined. So there is a real gap, a sort of vacuum in the leadership of nursing.

In addition to uncertainty about new roles and responsibilities, one study respondent, a nurse, observed that even where new roles are now in operation, there is uncertainty about their cost-effectiveness and therefore their long-term viability.

Conceptualizing the basis of uncertainty: ideas in conflict

Uncertainty about professional identity as discussed in the preceding chapter, together with the uncertainty in relation to risk from patients and in relation to training and leadership strategies for new roles as discussed in this chapter, can all be read as symptoms of more general contradictions faced by nurses.

In her influential book *Gender and the Professional Predicament in Nursing*, together with a paper published a year later in *Sociology*, Davies (1995, 1996a) sets out an analysis of the contradictions that nurses face. A key point in her analysis is the tension she notes between nurses' allegiance to 'profession', an idea to which she – following others, including Glaser and Slater (1987) – attributes the qualities of objectivity, competition, individualism, monopoly and mystique (Davies 1996a: 669), and the central value of 'care'. On the one hand, nurses are committed to ideas about profession and a process of professionalization. This process, as she points out, is not undifferentiated but is one which offers different routes including 'new professionalism' and democratic professionalism (p. 673). On the other hand, there is the idea of care and its centrality to an understanding of what nurses do. Associated with the idea of caring are ideas about relatedness, connectedness and intersubjectivity.

A further key point in Davies's argument is her observation of the difficulties incurred when an occupational group is 'ordered to care' in a patriarchal culture which does not value caring. Davies suggests that the work of nursing is in distinct contradiction to the notion of profession. She notes how professional concern keeps emotion at a distance. 'Professionals offer a detached "understanding" when clients, in what can be a highly charged context, frequently apologise for their fears and their tears' (Davies 1996a: 670). These attributes, she argues, are masculinist as indeed is the claim to autonomy. She writes: 'autonomy stands at the very heart of both cultural concepts of masculinity and of professions' (p. 670), and goes on to explain how one individual's autonomy requires considerable work on the part of others. She gives the example of the hospital consultant:

> Take for example the appearance of the hospital consultant in the outpatient department or on the ward round. This involves a direct encounter with the patient, but it is a *fleeting encounter*. It is sustained through bureaucratic recording systems that are the work of others, through much preparatory and often considerable follow-up work with patients by others. It is only through this activity that the work can take on its active, agentic and distant and controlling character. Autonomy therefore turns out to require considerable additional work without which it cannot be sustained.
>
> (p. 670)

Davies makes the important observation that women seeking change in the world of work are asking for inclusion in a system of relations already predicated on their work, for example as secretaries, nurses, junior hospital doctors. It is only when we grasp this fact that alternative forms of organization might make a difference. Davies notes how market philosophies and forms of managerialism have recently presented a particularly effective challenge to professional hegemony, together with consumer rhetoric of client empowerment (p. 673). As I understand it, there is a hint within her broad analysis that contradictions might be reconciled if nurses were to reject profession and to embrace aspects of consumerism such as the idea of consumer empowerment.

Certainly, care together with compassion and a concern for the common good are values in tension with competition, self-interest and objectivity. However, there is more than one way of conceptualizing the tension. Davies tends to privilege the negative attributes of profession (for example, self-interest and competition) over the altruistic (such as care and compassion). And she privileges the positive attributes of consumer or enterprise culture (for example, client empowerment) over the potentially negative (such as the surveillance of nurses and other health professionals by patients). A cursory reading of her analysis might, as noted above, lead one to suppose that she concludes that nurses should reject the idea of profession. Yet Davies does not appear to reject the idea of profession outright. She acknowledges fairly recent reappraisals of the idea of profession, notably the work of Hugman (1991) and Stacey (1992). Both authors are committed to shaping a new vision of professionalism, one which is inclusive of the influence of clients and users of services. Davies's main concern lies with the masculinist values of 'old professionalism' which is under attack for its 'monopolistic tendencies and inward-looking character' (Davies 1995: 137).

Davies's analysis undeniably constitutes a major contribution towards understanding nursing's 'professional' predicament. However, there is one aspect of her argument which is puzzling, and that is the assumption, reflected at least in the formation of her argument, about the positive role of the market – consumerism in particular – in providing a way forward for nursing. The findings upon which this present book is predicated – both literature sources and respondents' interviews – suggest a rather different perspective. It is agreed that a needs-led service should prevail over inflexible role demarcations. However, as noted in Chapter 3, moves to dislodge professional power are not evenly applied across all professional groups, and there is a danger that nurses will lose rather than gain ground in the so-called democratic reforms to the professions. In the field of health care, enterprise culture has made little difference to the power relationship between medicine and nursing, and nurses sense this despite the 'talking up nursing' that comes from nursing leaders. As underlined throughout the book, professional identity appears to matter. Where professional identity is challenged, demoralization and a sense of diminished confidence may, in turn, adversely affect the care given and compassion shown to patients. Its erosion should be a matter of concern to consumers of care, nurses, doctors and policy makers alike.

The need to address how uncertainty can inspire rather than threaten innovation in primary care is critical. The shape and substance of new and innovative nursing roles will depend on the ideas used to justify them, and our findings suggest that there is a balance to be struck between enterprise and profession. In the currently changing climate, ideas associated with enterprise and the market have tended to take precedence, as we have implied. How far these will be moderated by Labour's call (as expressed in the recent White Papers) for collaboration, integration and a statutory duty for National Health Service trusts to work in partnership with other National Health Service organizations remains to be seen. Certainly, not all aspects of the market appear to be rejected, as reflected in statements like 'the Government wants to keep what has worked about fundholding' (Department of Health 1998: 3). As already noted, it is unlikely that competition and self-interest will entirely cease to influence health care provision. Therefore it is important that nursing leaders and other health care policy makers continue to acknowledge factors which may undermine a clear, confident nursing contribution to primary health care.

5 Exploiting the potential for innovation in primary care

How can the present uncertainties in primary health care inspire rather then threaten innovation? One of the conclusions to be drawn from Chapter 4 is that innovation rests at least in part on striking a balance between enterprise culture, together with its associated values, and the need for a sense of professional identity. This chapter is about the implications of this conclusion for innovation in primary care, especially in relation to the role of primary care nursing.

It is important to recognize that nurses will differ in their views about the potential for innovation in primary care. Undoubtedly there are a number of potential avenues for innovation in primary care nursing. Referring to a study evening on the menopause and hormone replacement therapy, a practice nurse in the NPCRDC study reported how, while initially feeling alarmed at being the only nurse there, she was heartened to find that her knowledge was on a par with the doctors who included a consultant obstetrician and gynaecologist. Reflecting on the shift in her areas of work, she presented a real sense of gaining ground, saying 'I've got a few patients and I've actually built up good relationships . . . which has been quite satisfying to me because he [the general practitioner] has been quite happy to accept that – to hand them over to me – and to take my advice, you know. And that is something I feel I've achieved.' However, she appended these remarks with the words, 'I think you've got to be careful how extended this role is because at the end of the day nurses are nurses, and they are trained to be just nurses.' Her words can be read in a number of ways. They reflect a degree of certainty about role and professional identity and, indeed, nurse/ patient relationships. The word 'just' in her final phrase is interesting and hints at how the nurse viewed her status against that of the general practitioners with whom she was working.

The practice nurse's words stand in some contrast to the following example of more assertive expressions of growth, enterprise and the potential for innovation. Another practice nurse, interviewed in late 1996, commented:

'with nurses, there would be nothing to stop them setting up their own practices should the imminent Primary Health Care Bill make the changes many nurses are hoping for.' The idea of nurses setting up primary care practices is innovative; however, a more radical view of the potential for innovation is apparent in a debate which is gathering momentum around the idea that the nurse practitioner role represents an 'evolving and discrete professional group, outside the currently accepted professional and occupational definitions of nursing and medicine' (Barton *et al.* 1999). The authors who put forward this idea base their analysis on their experiences of running a nurse practitioner undergraduate programme. They assert that 'there can be no question that the diagnosis made by a nurse practitioner is a medical one, complemented and enhanced by a parallel nursing one' (p. 61).

Inevitably, new roles will emerge and they will be challenged. As suggested in Chapter 2, the challenge will likely be around the issue of cost-effectiveness, an issue which has slowed down innovation in the past, as was the case with nurse practitioners in Canada following Spitzer *et al.*'s 1974 study. Recent UK studies have evaluated amongst other factors (Clement *et al.* 1999; Kinnersley *et al.* 2000) the cost effectiveness of nurse practitioners (Venning *et al.* 2000). Venning *et al.'s* study concludes that if nurse practitioners were able to maintain the benefits (patient satisfaction, low start up costs) while shortening consultation times they 'could be more cost-effective than general practitioners' (p. 1048). This cautious but, nevertheless, positive finding is broadly welcomed by nurses and general practitioners who have been afraid that the nurse practitioner role in primary care will be shown not to be cost-effective in spite of local knowledge of better outcomes for patients. The tension here between different points of view echoes in some respects Alford's (1975: xiv) point that health care institutions can be understood in terms of a continuing struggle between competing interests. Alford describes the situation in the USA some twenty-five years ago as one where powerful and strategically located interests effectively resisted change, and, to crudely summarize his argument, studies of the health care system actually became part of the system to be understood. While I would not want to suggest that contemporary UK studies of the cost-effectiveness of new and changing nursing roles represent powerful, vested interests, Alford reminds us that cost-effectiveness is a contested issue.

Contested issues notwithstanding, challenges to innovation in nursing can be viewed as healthy. Whether or not new roles are 'effective' matters to a profession concerned with providing a service to the public, whatever the definition of effectiveness. In their discussion of the effectiveness of teamworking in primary health care, West and Slater (1996) observe that there remains considerable confusion about the concept of effectiveness. The authors offer a useful analysis of existing literature on organizational effectiveness noting the distinction made between effectiveness (doing the right thing) and efficiency (doing things right) and stressing that conceptual as well as empirical development in evaluating the effectiveness of primary health care is urgent (p. 28). This is an area where nurses could usefully participate, and one which would help the profession to identify areas of strength in its provision of an effective and efficient service as well as one which is caring and compassionate.

Certainly, the shape and substance of new and changing primary care roles will depend on the ideas and values used to justify them. Compassion does not necessarily preclude a degree of self-interest, and without self-interest confidence may falter and nurses might retreat into a particularly negative form of profession. The strength of a nursing contribution to innovation in primary care rests on a profession with confidence in its ability to make a significant difference to the provision of health care. Confidence is the key to transforming uncertainty into action and innovation. By this I mean a careful, considered confidence in the recognition that nurses may, in certain circumstances, lead multidisciplinary efforts to provide better health outcomes for patients. In the remainder of this chapter, I review two overlapping preconditions for moving forward such an agenda. These are, first, an education which prepares nurses for the tasks they face and where it is recognized that compassion requires competence; and second, a climate which fosters collaboration and teamwork across professional groups. The chapter concludes with a discussion of the areas of primary care where nursing can most usefully lead in the provision of better health outcomes for patients.

Preconditions for innovation: educating and preparing nurses for primary health care

Almost without exception all fifteen interviewees on the NPCRDC study commented on the education and preparation of primary care nurses, despite the absence of an initial lead question on the topic by the interviewer. The two key themes emerging from discussion are (1) the current status of nurse education, and (2) the need to make good certain deficits in nurse education, specifically in relation to training primary care nurses to confront and deal with uncertainty. Underpinning the two themes is a general recognition of the importance of an understanding of the status of nursing care and its contribution in the wider context of the delivery of multidisciplinary health care.

The current status of nurse education

As Witz (1992) usefully summarizes, there is a new philosophy of nursing: one which attempts to replace a routinized, task-orientated approach with one that is problem-solving and patient-centred. This philosophy has been the driver for change in nurse education for at least twenty years, and the basis for the acceleration of change through the Project 2000 initiative in the 1990s. In the view of one study respondent, by and large the changes in education spearheaded by Project 2000 have made a difference. She noted in interview:

> I think at long last nurses are becoming more aware of all these issues [evidence-based practice, relationship between doctors and nurses, economics of care] and I think this is the product of a better education. Now, OK, it's very patchy, we know there's criticism of many courses. But by and large, slowly but surely, I think education is beginning to make a difference.

Elaborating on the difference she commented:

> We are seeing it in more critical kinds of reviews in the journals. The [Nursing] Times and the [Nursing] Standard have some quite good commentary in them now. I think the editors are tuned into this – that nurses no longer want to be spoon fed; that nurses are quite capable of reading some critical commentary on things.

And she noted how this critical commentary was motivating student nurses and qualified nurses to look at their own practice so that:

> Trusts are now saying 'we really know the difference when it's your graduates coming on the wards'. Maybe they are trying to butter us up, but the students have had four years of good education and if they can't make a difference then we shouldn't be running the course.

Part of the difference the students were making was a knock-on effect where, as the respondent explained, 'the qualified nurses at first feel defensive because they feel they are way behind these young people, but, you know, they then do come on courses with us'. Atkins and Williams (1994) hint similarly in a paper which reports on a study exploring the relationships between undergraduate nursing students and their non-graduate health visiting mentors in practice. Common to both the respondent's comments and the study reported by Atkins and Williams is the finding that nurses feel the need for an education which offers breadth and depth of understanding on the issues which confront them in daily practice. For our respondent, it was about 'understanding where our patients are coming from – how age, race, gender, class and geographical location will determine why they are ill in the first place, and something of the ability of nurses to respond in a positive way.' She added that 'if nurses do not understand and do not respond, they have no business being nurses.' Reflecting on her own preparation for nursing in the 1950s she explained:

> I was a gold medallist. I reckon I was a very good nurse. I practised holistic care as far as I was able. I certainly thought we were holistic in

the sense that we did everything for our patients, literally, including giving them their meals and feeding them if they couldn't feed themselves, etc., taking them to the toilet and washing them afterwards, and measuring their urine and keeping them on fluid charts, answering in the fear of death to the ward sister if they [the fluid charts] hadn't been maintained properly throughout the day. I think in that sense we were very good nurses. What we lacked – what I felt the loss of terribly – was an education. I loved the people. That's why I stayed in nursing actually. I knew from virtually day one that it [nursing] was not going to stimulate me intellectually – but I was lucky being able to buy into that at a later stage.

The respondent's comments were made in the context of a discussion about what nursing skills may have been lost as a result of a move from the apprenticeship system prior to Project 2000. As such, they anticipate current concerns prompted by the Secretary of State's pronouncement in 1999, referred to in Chapter 3, that nurse education might be misplaced within the higher education sector. However, unlike concerns about nurses' alleged loss of practical skills and loss of National Health Service involvement in nurse education (Lawson 1999; Secretary of State 1999), there is no appeal to a romantic past in nursing. The respondent also anticipated concern about changing workforce expectations. Just as she once felt the lack of an education so now nurses expect one. Amongst the key issues for the United Kingdom Central Council Education Committee, as suggested by Warner *et al.* (1998), is the issue of changing workforce expectations. This issue is closely linked to the other key issues cited in their report *Healthcare Futures 2010*. They are the demographic facts of an increasing population of older people, more diseases of old age, increasing levels of disability from mental illness, new genetic approaches, increasing requirements for evidence-based practice, more care outside district general hospitals, new forms of information transfer, and changing professional roles between and within professions. It is quite difficult to imagine how one would educate nurses to make an informed contribution to this kind of agenda without educating them within the higher education sector, for reasons such as those offered by the respondent. She noted, referring to undergraduate students:

Nurses now have greater opportunities to expand their thinking, to have a rationale for understanding why they are doing what they are doing, and for actually having a base from which they can argue for certain things, both for patients and for themselves – because they have learned in a broader sense what we learned as student nurses – and we are giving them, slowly but surely, the tools to be more equal.

She was well aware of the likely challenges to a thinking breed of nurse, noting that some might not be willing or able to accept that nurses should think and argue on an equal footing with doctors. She continued:

Now if the doctors aren't able to accept that yet and take that on – in a way it's their problem. I do think those changes are very evident and I see it amongst nurses in practice just as much as nurses in academia. I think it's the medics who haven't bothered – because they have always been so privileged – to take on this massive change in thinking, culture and orientation that is permeating nursing now, and therefore they are just sitting there and thinking they don't have to change. But I think the weight of the scales is slowly but surely building up.

Managers, however, were more of a concern:

The unknown quantity is the extent to which the health care manager who is such a key player now in terms of budget control, will continue to believe that actually it is the doctor who will deliver what he wants as a manager, and that the nurse can continue to be discounted.

These words remind us that what might be seen as a gain from a nursing perspective could be viewed as negative from a workforce management perspective, as discussed in Chapter 3 in connection with the report *The Future Healthcare Workforce* (Health Services Management Unit 1996). Early in 1999, the Secretary of State chose to note that the move of nursing into the higher education sector was likely a cause of nursing shortages. His argument rested on what he perceived to be the 'virtual withdrawal of Health Service involvement' from nurse education and concerns that young people might be put off by 'the nature of the course' (Secretary of State for Health 1999). His comments prompted varying responses which included those who broadly supported his point of view, if not in every detail (Lawson 1999; Lilley 1999; Phillips 1999). Common to the voices of support for the Secretary for State were ideas about nurses not needing a degree or diploma to nurse, although none said fully what they meant by nursing. Certainly one does not need a degree to give a bedpan but then neither does one need a degree to do many of the things doctors do. The point is that tasks like giving bedpans, taking blood pressure – tasks laypeople can and do undertake – are only part of nursing or medical schemes of care. These are schemes which require an ability to undertake many other highly skilled tasks of course. Importantly, they also require an ability to interpret and assess complex situations and symptoms;to make difficult decisions which affect many other people's lives and health; and to justify these decisions to one's colleagues and defend them, if necessary, in law. These skills require knowledge and experience. In medicine – a relatively recent arrival in higher education when compared with, say, philosophy – basic knowledge has been acquired in the laboratory, tutorials and in the lecture hall. Practical experience only really commences in the house year as many a sister and staff nurse can confirm. In nursing, the expectation has been that nurses must somehow know it all on the day they start work as staff nurses. This expectation was as unrealistic with the apprenticeship system prior to Project 2000 as it is today, and nurse educators are concerned to explore schemes of preceptorship as a means of consolidating the knowledge and experience gained as a student. However, these schemes are virtually impossible to operate in a health service short of around 13,000 nurses (cf. Rafferty 1999).

Nursing will continue to have to strenuously defend its right to access higher education. As already noted, not only is it the case that higher education is a critical factor in the nursing profession's ability to deliver high quality care in a primary care-led National Health Service but also, and importantly, nursing can make a difference to higher education insofar as it allows for the entry of an increased number of students, mainly women, often with non-traditional qualifications (for example, those pursuing post-registration degrees and other courses). Nursing's entry into universities is in this way a major contribution towards the feminization and democratization of those institutions (Howard 1999; Martin 1999; Rafferty 1999). As one of the study's respondents put it: 'we must never lose sight of the gender issue for any of the professions, because women have to make sure they get as good an education as men . . . I really see that as one of the great hopes for the future. I just hope they don't take it off us . . . and put us all back in hospitals, as I'm sure many of the consortia [health service-led groups who purchase nurse training] would like to do.'

There is a strong case to be made for retaining nurse education in the higher education sector. There are, however, ways in which education could and should be improved, including the need for providers of nurse education to be more responsive to service needs. As one respondent commented in late 1996, 'I think nursing departments in universities are being pushed by people like me and by other people saying if you don't start delivering care – moving towards the clinical area – then you won't get the money; if you don't provide the kind of nurses we need then we'll just pull the plug and say we'll go elsewhere.' The need for universities to be more responsive to service needs is acknowledged in the government's new strategy for educating and training nurses. The *Times Higher Education Supplement* (1999: 4) reports that a key feature of the new system will be stronger and more effective working relationships between the National Health Service and the universities. According to the report, the strategy is welcomed by the Royal College of Nursing and by the Committee of Vice Chancellors, the latter commenting that 'universities endorse a partnership approach and are working closely with the local National Health Service Trust hospitals and community services'.

Training for uncertainty

We now turn to the second theme for discussion, the need to make good certain deficits in nurse education, specifically training primary care nurses to confront and deal with uncertainty.

Three factors have been identified which contribute towards a culture of uncertainty: the erosion of professional identity, risk in relation to patients, and uncertainty in relation to new roles. One way of addressing uncertainty is to reduce it. In relation to professional identity, as noted by Williams and Sibbald (1999: 744), policy makers and managers need to be aware that further erosion of professional boundaries may lead to greater uncertainty and low staff morale. In addressing uncertainty in relation to patients, attention should be paid to the legal infrastructure which enables nurses to undertake tasks formerly undertaken by general practitioners. Considerable thought has already been given to the legal position of nurse prescribing. This could be extended to other areas, including liability and negligence. In addressing uncertainty in relation to role at the local level, practices supporting workforce changes require distinctions between professional roles to enable more efficient exploitation of current opportunities. It would therefore seem appropriate for individual contracts to be used where nurses assume new roles. These would provide clarity regarding boundaries with other health care professionals, combined with security to avoid exploitation and overlap (Williams *et al.* 1997). At a more global level, Barton *et al.* (1999) suggest the formal recording of qualifications, for example 'nurse practitioner' on the professional register. However, as the authors point out, 'another, and more likely, possibility is the recording of nurse practitioner status within a specialist practice framework'. This, they claim, 'would bring at least some professional endorsement and protection of the title' (p. 62).

The recommendations noted are based on the desire to give greater clarity, indeed certainty, to the current situation, and they are important principally in the short term. In a context where patient safety and well-being are paramount, it would seem appropriate to take this line of argument. Even so, it is not always possible to provide clarity in respect of the wider health care context – including interprofessional relationships and nurse/patient relationships – in all situations and at all times. Thought could, therefore, also be directed to more radical changes in the culture of nursing: towards an effort to accept, confront and manage uncertainties. Indeed, as the following words of a study respondent convey, nurses are turning their thoughts to the need for such change.

> Doctors' training from the very beginning teaches them about uncertainty – they are trained for uncertainty – whereas we are not. We are never prepared for uncertainty. What we have then is a profession that is very frightened and wants somebody to give them a piece of paper to say I've been trained to do this – so they want a piece of paper that covers every single thing they're going to be asked to do, which is not your average generic nursing. And I mean it is so limiting really, when what you really need is a profession that is autonomous enough and confident enough to be able to recognize the limits of their own competence and their own boundaries.

What might training for uncertainty include? As already suggested, nurses need to be aware of the various factors that affect them as a profession so that insecurity and uncertainty are not seen as simply personal failure. It is important to understand the nature of the uncertainties faced by nurses. Inclusion of sociology and social policy in the curriculum go some way to illuminating the uncertainties as, according to Giddens (1986), no social processes are unalterable laws, and as human beings we are not condemned to be swept along by forces that have the inevitability of laws of nature (p. 22). As nursing is swept along by the tide of rapid change in society and in health care we can turn to the sociological imagination to help us understand what is happening to us. Sociology can help us to take a hand in controlling our own destinies (Williams *et al.* 1998: xiii).

It is also important to include in the curricula the practical skills and the scientific knowledge that nurses need to support new roles. For example, nurse practitioners need diagnostic skills and the knowledge to underpin new skills (Jordan 1994). It is also essential for nurses to recognize the possibility of alternative 'diagnoses' or assessments of patients, recognition which is integrated into doctors' thinking. For nursing, this might involve training in the utilization of alternative strategies in the management of care and a heightening of awareness of the various risk factors associated with each. Realization that there is not necessarily an immediately correct diagnosis or assessment is important. In a recent study exploring changing roles and identities in primary care nursing, as yet not completed, a mock objective structured clinical examination (OSCE) – the process by which the students' diagnostic skills are assessed – was held for nurse practitioner students. In the discussion with medical colleagues during the debriefing which followed, the issue of how to deal with 'not being sure of a diagnosis', even with increased pathophysiology training, was discussed. Some of the doctors present congratulated a nurse practitioner student on her examination of a patient and on her interpretation and management of the situation. Understanding that the doctors present found the processes of diagnosis difficult appeared liberating for some of the students. Hearing the doctors present saying that they would not necessarily have made the same diagnosis, nor would theirs necessarily be the more correct, was quite a learning curve for the nurses present in accepting and dealing with uncertainty. It was an example, as yet all too infrequent, of a positive learning encounter between nurses and doctors where the topic of discussion is equally critical to both parties. There appeared to be no attempt to talk down from either the doctors or nurses present. Indeed, there was more of a sense of engagement between the two professional groups than is sometimes the case *within* each group.

Fostering interprofessional collaboration and teamwork

The need for collaboration and teamwork in primary care was a key theme to emerge from the NPCRDC study data. All respondents appealed to the idea of teamwork in one way or another. Given their interest in primary health care, this finding is not surprising. Teamwork in primary care has been the subject of research for at least a decade, both within the UK (Bond *et al.* 1985; West and Wallace 1991; Wiles and Robinson 1994; Wood *et al.* 1994; West and Field 1995; Long 1996) and outside the UK for example, in the USA (Jones 1992) and Spain (Peiro *et al.* 1992). Within the broad context of teamwork, the critical issue for many study respondents was the issue of shared learning.

The issue of shared learning

In the words of one study respondent, 'if we don't get nurse education right – if we want primary care teams to work properly and to deliver a primary care-led National Health Service which is health based – then we have to train them, we actually have to make sure that all training should be interprofessional – there should be no uni-profession'. She continued with the following questions:

Why are we training practice nurses and nurse practitioners separately from GPs? Why are we training social workers and others separately from nurses and the other people they are working with? For me the only way forward is to have shared learning. The second thing is to make sure the people who teach nurses – the nurse educators – actually should have to practice and should be aware of what working in a team is about. Because most of them never work in teams. They work in separate departments in a university, don't they?

The respondent's questions raise a number of issues in respect of the idea of shared learning. First, her words are fairly radical insofar as she is promoting here at least the possibility of a common entrance to health and social care studies which would include medicine; that is if one reads her words as relating to *basic* medicine, nursing, social work and other professions' schemes of education. Wicks (1998) suggests a more radical spin on this idea of shared learning. The solution for 'working together' from Wicks's point of view, is a fundamental restructuring of the health workforce. In particular, she proposes 'doctors be nurses'. By this she means that aspiring doctors ought first to undertake a degree in nursing. She elaborates her proposal as follows:

This should be a degree with elements of both arts and science and with a strong emphasis on an ecological and holistic approach to health and illness, health education, public and community health, as well as the clinical theory, experience and skills required. After a year's practice as nurses, graduates could then choose to continue to work with their present qualification (as a first rung or generic health worker) or go on to postgraduate studies in nursing (clinical or community), complementary modalities, medicine, public health or other specialisms. In this way it would be possible to retain the effective aspects of modern medicine, integrated with a perspective which emphasises holism, illness prevention and the relationships between health, illness, individual life history and social structure.

(Wicks 1998: 181)

While radical, her suggestions are not as far-fetched as they might at first appear. Depending on one's perspective, the proposal she puts forward is a marked improvement on the scheme as suggested by Schofield and colleagues (Health Services Management Unit 1996) – a scheme which does not include medicine in its proposal for a generic workforce. As Wicks notes, there is a worldwide trend to changing medical degrees to postgraduate education. This is reflected in the burgeoning of degrees, at undergraduate level, in medical humanities or health sciences, that offer a route into postgraduate studies in medicine, nursing and other health-related areas. The radical element of Wicks's proposal is that nursing becomes a prerequisite for all aspiring health care workers, whether they progress to nursing, medicine or other health professions. While there may be some conceptual and operational difficulties, the proposal has merit insofar as it suggests that 'unless all health care workers including doctors (by virtue of undertaking the common basic education) are prepared to touch and lift and clean and dress, as well as examine and prescribe and treat' (p. 181), they will not succeed in their respective careers.

There are caveats which could be usefully applied to Wicks's proposal, not least that rigorous standards are set and monitored in respect of the care given by those in training for 'first rung or generic health care worker', and the question of who is to do this has to be answered. Many patients will undoubtedly benefit from the exposure of medical students and others to the tasks listed. Indeed, medical students are currently exposed through vacation work as health care assistants. However, as we know from the number of nurses who go before professional disciplinary committees, exposure of health care workers to undertaking 'basic' care does not guarantee compassion and proper conduct (Williams 2000). From an educational perspective, there would likely be logistical problems around pitching the standard of entry qualifications. While it might have some benefits, a common foundation to all health care work does not remove questions about who should do what in, for example, primary health care, and who makes decisions about who should do what. However, Wicks hints at how the relationship between medicine and nursing might be changed insofar as her proposal offers the possibility of a shared common foundation curriculum, and thus the possibility of mutual understandings of health issues. Shared learning in the early years might well address some of the problems experienced by those who are currently trying to bring the different professionals together to learn to work in teams, as reflected in the discussion below.

Returning to the idea that, if we want primary care teams to work then training should be interdisciplinary, the issue of teamwork raised by the nurse respondent in the NPCRDC study intersects with findings from other studies. For example, West and Slater (1996: 29) flag the lack of pre-qualification teamworking training for professionals in primary care and note how this has adversely affected health care delivery. Despite recognition that shared learning is important, it became apparent in the NPCRDC study that shared learning continues to be a vexed issue. One study respondent, a general practitioner, recounted his experiences of trying to encourage teamwork by bringing together nurses and general practitioner trainees for workshops on topics of mutual interest:

> I was probably one of the first course organizers in the country to put district nurse students and the GP trainees together on a day release course. We [a lecturer in district nursing and the GP] brought together nurses and the GP trainees in an area where we thought they would have common ground, like terminal care . . . We put health visitors and GP trainees together in areas where we thought they might have common ground, like child abuse, and all they did was fight, constantly.

He continued:

> It seems that they [nurses] had attitudes about working with GPs even before they developed any team experience of their own, and it seemed also that these were the attitudes of the people that taught them . . . I think we really need to start them off a lot earlier, and I think that teachers need very careful selection too. When we tried again, the GP trainees rebelled, refused to meet with the district nurses . . . This was only a couple of months ago . . . then we tried again on a day release course and they formed two separate groups like young people at a dance, and wouldn't talk to each other.

The respondent here alludes to attitudes on the part of nursing which might act as a barrier to teamwork. When prompted, he ventured that nurses had appeared defensive. In the light of the findings in relation to uncertainty about role and professional identity, perhaps this is not surprising. Another respondent, a nurse, suggested that a potential barrier was medicine's absolute commitment to 'a science-based, medically oriented approach'. She had made efforts to get doctors and nurses together to discuss moral, ethical and resource issues, but had met with resistance by doctors who, from her perspective, did not see how these issues might touch on both professions and that shared discussion might throw light on these topics. A general practitioner suggested that a barrier to teamwork between doctors and nurses could be the individualism that is encouraged by medical education. She noted in respect of junior doctors a tendency 'towards being an extrovert rather than someone who says "that won't be for the good of the team", or "the good of the unit".' She added, 'I don't think we make enough of teamwork – if junior doctors knew they were being judged on their team skills rather than their ability to cope in a crisis, then maybe they would pay

more attention – perhaps that would make a difference.' This general practitioner also alluded to structural barriers relating to sex. She noted the
predominance of women in medicine in Russia, adding:

> The women in Russia are not valued, they are not well paid. Here [UK],
> what I see going on is a number of largely female doctors working
> extremely well with nurses doing a lot of good stuff for patients, but
> they are represented by men in national committees who are not . . . who
> are quite arrogant and ignorant and who probably don't relate terribly
> well with their nursing colleagues at the top. I don't know if there is
> any evidence about this, but one way or another we have some difficulty
> in how we are going to deal with these people at the top.

She went on to make a further interesting point about sex, race and teamwork:

> What we want is people working together, shoulder to shoulder, not
> doctors leaving a team of nurses while he spins off and plays golf or
> something. And nurses aren't the only subservient group. There are
> women [GPs] who are treated as somehow second rate from the prin-
> cipals – especially non-white women. They are dumped on quite often
> and we have to protect them as well as nurses. Indeed, the subservient
> woman doctor has only the GMC [General Medical Council] to go to,
> whereas if you get a nurse who is put upon she can actually go to the
> nursing union and she is relatively in the stronger position.

Structural difficulties were an issue amongst respondents, both nurses and
doctors. Another general practitioner respondent went on to explain how
teams would 'never really function as long as you have two modes of
employment, where the general practitioners are independent contractors
and the nurses employed in a hierarchical system or indeed the employees
of general practitioners.' In the longer term he felt:

> The way of doing this – getting teams to work effectively – is, and this
> depends on your political persuasion, they are either all salaried or all
> independent contractors with nurses coming together with doctors (like
> GP principals in partnership) as nurse partners, contributing to the
> financial income perhaps and drawing from it in exactly the same way
> as general practitioners do. Then you would have people motivated to
> work in partnership – in a team rather than what is at present a situ-
> ation of divided loyalties partly towards management and partly towards
> the practice – and there's often tension between these for the nurses.

Both general practitioners' observations on the structural aspects of the
nurse/doctor relationship are helpful and confirm findings from other studies (West and Slater 1996). From the latter general practitioner's perspective, real engagement depends on changing the system in the way he suggests.
He was talking in late 1996 and saw tasks or work changing for both doctors
and nurses, but felt that the relationship between doctors and nurses had

little chance of changing, although he was keen to assert that, on a different and more personal level, nurses, as is the case with general practitioners, develop areas of expertise for which they are respected by both doctors and nurses alike. He said, 'GPs have different limits in a partnership, you know. Someone refers frequently in one area and not another and vice versa. And so for nurses. And it's not always a matter of education, you know, but how you feel about someone you work with.' Other respondents hinted at this kind of relationship. One practice nurse spoke of how a nurse practitioner was treated as an 'absolute equal in the practice'. She said, 'if she does a travel vaccination, they give her the income, she's done it, prescribed it and everything. She gets the income for that particular consultation.'

However, one nursing respondent believed strongly that personal recognition by other health professionals was a poor substitute for partnership. She commented that new realms of nursing work are being achieved 'by grace and favour', and continued:

> I believe, in nursing, the closer you get to the doctor, and the closer the relationship you have, the more you think you've gained, because what you've gained is the GP or the principal's trust. And that means a lot to a nurse – being trusted, being valued, their opinion counted, having a referral accepted, having a doctor sign a blank prescription. And the pity is that if it is power, it is really a very delegated power. The best analogy I can think of is the traditional husband/wife syndrome. The way it works best in primary care is where the practice nurse is the doctor's wife – then you have everything – ultimate trust.

Her words, together with the general practitioner's, reflect the view that for collaboration and teamwork to be effective, a radical shift in the power relationship is required. If hierarchies are to be flattened as Schofield and his colleagues (Health Services Management Unit 1996) suggest then they should be flattened evenly across medicine and nursing. This said, one general practitioner had the following remarks to make in relation to getting teams to work together effectively:

> Until teams begin to look at the whole range of problems that patients bring to the practice, not only patients but carers too, and we *all* begin to talk about what's best done by nurses and what's best done by GPs . . . Say, someone with terminal illness – unless we ask the questions *with the patients, with their carers, with groups of patients*, what's best done by a GP? What can only be done by a GP? What can only be done by a nurse? Until you begin to address questions like that you won't move forward.

His words anticipated the mood for partnership that has become a feature of changes enshrined in the policies around the change in government in 1997. To reiterate, in recent years, policy initiatives and organizational changes within the National Health Service have created a strong impulse for rethinking the role played by nurses in multidisciplinary approaches towards the provision of improved health care (Richardson and Maynard 1995). The key drivers for change (the issue of cost-effectiveness and a declining recruitment to the general practitioner workforce) are intimately linked with concerns about rebuilding public confidence in the National Health Service (Department of Health 1998) and with a commitment to a health service which is responsive to 'the needs, expectations and experiences of patients' (Welsh Office 1998a: chapter 3). The route to such a health service is now seen to be achieved through collaboration and partnership at national and local levels both across professional and service boundaries and across boundaries between patients and providers of care (Department of Health 1998; Welsh Office 1998a).

The patient's point of view

Thus, a key challenge at local level is to put in place a system which will gauge the patient's point of view and which will allow for collaboration between professionals and patients. As reflected in the general practitioner's words cited earlier, an understanding of lay assessments of care is critical. 'Patients' perceptions are important, not only because they are a barometer of the appropriateness and effectiveness of services, but because they are a unique source of knowledge about the way in which people use services when they do for the reasons that they do' (Rogers and Elliott 1997: 59). In using services, patients enter into relationships with primary care professionals. These relationships are poorly understood and nurses may wish to lead empirical investigations of the degree to which patients share professionals' understandings of issues of responsibility and accountability in primary care. This would begin to assist a better understanding of how to develop collaborative schemes which promote effective use of services, although the issue of how to resolve differences between patients' and professionals' perceptions would need to be addressed, as would the weight given to patients' perceptions against those of the professionals.

Research suggests there are areas of agreement as well as important differences between lay and professional conceptions of health and illness (see, for example, Cornwell 1986; Calnan and Williams 1992). For although doctors and nurses are strongly socialized into their respective roles, they share the commonly held ideas, values and expectations of the society of which they are a part. At the same time, patients have become increasingly knowledgeable about medical science, health promotion and health service delivery through formal education as well as exposure to media coverage of current health issues (Karpf 1988; Gabe *et al.* 1991). One might also expect to find correspondence, as well as differences, between lay and professional understandings of issues related to changing roles in health service provision.

For example, there may be agreement about the need for prompt access to a practitioner. However, there may be disagreement between professionals and patients about which practitioner is the most appropriate.

In respect of the latter point, there are, of course, variations between patients' views. As noted in Chapter 4, there is the view that what the nursing profession has to get to grips with is that patients do not necessarily worry about who does the task, what they want is the task done by a competent person. In some contrast, there is literature which suggests that patients want continuity of care with a specific professional (Sweeney and Gray 1995; Freeman and Richards 1993), and that some women may prefer to consult a woman (Brooks and Phillips 1996). Relatedly, there is evidence which suggests that female patients are more likely than male patients to prefer to see a nurse (Bond *et al.* 1998). There is also evidence to suggest a conservatism amongst older people for consulting with a nurse rather than a general practitioner (Bond *et al.* 1998). In an evaluation of nurse practitioners in Northumberland, it is suggested that 'a large majority' of patients are willing to consult with trained nurse practitioners, and that exposure to such consultations increases patients' willingness to consult again and with a wider range of problems (Bond *et al.* 1998). The study asserts that 'more patients view the consultations provided by TNPs [trained nurse practitioners] as more positive than those provided by general practitioners' (Bond *et al.* 1998: 59). However, the study does not appear to have interrogated the basis of the confidence expressed in any detail. For example, it did not investigate how an individual patient's views may also change in relation to different areas of primary care: namely health promotion, chronic conditions and acute primary care. While the problem of the fit between primary care professionals' and patients' assessments of new and changing roles is recognized as important in the current and changing organization of primary health care, there is, to date, no detailed, systematic, empirical investigation of the fit between professional and lay assessments of new and changing roles in relation to clinical, administrative, professional and legal responsibilities.

Better outcomes for patients

In theory, it would seem reasonable to suppose that patients will be the main beneficiaries of a coordinated, collaborative approach to health care provision. The National Health Services Management Executive (1993: para. 4.3) has linked the importance of teamworking to the best outcomes for patients, stating: 'The best and most cost-effective outcomes for patients and clients are achieved when professionals work together, learn together, engage in clinical audit of outcomes together, and generate innovation to ensure progress in practice and service.' However, West and Slater (1996) point out, the effects of multidisciplinary teamworking are mixed: some positive but others problematic. On the positive side, and in respect of outcomes for patients, West and Slater note that there is improved health delivery in terms of, for example, better detection, treatment, follow-up and outcome in hypertension (citing Adorian *et al.* 1990) and fewer operations (citing Jones 1992) as a result of families receiving team care. On the negative side, it is perhaps telling that the authors emphasize that their respondents, drawn from local organization teams, saw multidisciplinary teamworking as having made only moderate or little contribution to the effectiveness of primary care in relation to health promotion, disease prevention, health needs assessment and relationships with patients and the community (West and Slater 1996: 21–2).

In many respects West and Slater's findings are hardly surprising given the climate of uncertainty within which the imperative to give patients best and cost-effective outcomes is to be implemented. Uncertainties need to be addressed if such an innovative agenda is to move forward. To this should be added the proviso, now recognized by those charged with setting the agenda for future health care research (for example, Welsh Office 1998a, c), that patients must be an integral part of the collaborative effort at policy, operational management and grassroots levels. In this respect the following observation from one of our respondents is useful. Commenting on patient satisfaction scales, he suggested that whether or not patients feel there are benefits depends to some extent on the criteria used to measure their views. He noted how patient satisfaction depends to some extent on how patients experience existing relationships between patient and practitioner, and added:

> I think with regard to patient satisfaction, initially the outcomes will vary because some patients really want care with a certain professional. They will already have a relationship with one professional – say a doctor – and not the other – say a nurse. It doesn't really matter whether it's a doctor or nurse – it's the relationship that counts, and patients may have strong feelings for one particular professional. These attitudes, maybe prejudices, will resolve in time, as patients get used to changes.

He recalled how, in his practice, midwifery was a case in point. At one time he had forged strong relationships with his midwifery cases, then midwives had taken over and, in time, equally strong relationships were forged between the midwives and pregnant women. He added that it was important to gauge benefits for patients in varying ways, taking account of the importance of the individual relationships between patient and practitioner. However, it is also important to take into account the possibility that one professional group, because of its training and particular abilities, could offer a better outcome for patients than another professional group.

His words remind us that, in parallel with addressing current uncertainties and taking patients' views seriously, it is also important to have a sense of what improved or better outcomes for patients might be, and a sense of what the differential contribution of doctors and nurses might be in realizing these outcomes. Here we are specifically interested in primary care nursing. Looking across our respondents' comments in this respect, the following themes predominate: first, improved continuity of care, and second, the possibility of benefits which might follow from rethinking the current conception of primary care as a first contact reactive service.

Improved continuity of care

In making a case for improved continuity of care, respondents stressed the complexity of factors involved. The suggestion that nurses are eminently suited to providing continuity of care, particularly in certain areas of care, came from general practitioners, nurses and the consumer spokesperson within the study. However, continuity of care was not seen unproblematically as the domain of nursing. Indeed, there were some concerns that the substitution of doctors for nurses disrupts continuity of care, in relation to both general practitioners' and nurses' work, and that it might undermine the two professions' relationships with patients. It is noted in Chapter 3 how the process of substitution has, for some general practitioners, eroded their capacity to care for families holistically. Where nurses are now undertaking the care of certain family members, for example a child who has diabetes, the general practitioner's view of the 'whole family' is disrupted, according to some general practitioners. One respondent suggested that general practitioners feel threatened by nurses, noting how, in her experience, 'they are worried that practice nurses are actually taking away from them their role of continuing care management of the chronically ill – asthmatics, diabetics – and they're only seeing people when there is a crisis.' She added, 'GPs say they don't actually like working in that way because they lose the sense of continuity with a patient.' Substitution was also seen to disrupt aspects of work seen by many to be central to a nursing role: namely, the 'everyday, basic continuity of what matters to patients'. One nurse respondent expressed great concern that 'there are people who are starving to death because nobody is feeding them, and trained nurses no longer feel that feeding patients is part of their role.' She added, 'primary care nurses at the moment – a lot of them – have lost their understanding of primary care – as prevention, continuity and attending to basic needs, you know.'

This observation notwithstanding, the point was made by another nurse that 'nurses do have a feel for something much broader in terms of what the delivery of humane care is about.' She said: 'I think this is because they are the people who spend most time with patients. The nurse has to sort of live part of her life with that patient's consciousness.' Another nurse's words throw some light on ideas about continuity of care, meeting basic needs and 'living with the patient's consciousness.' She referred to what she called 'the cup of tea issue' in relation to district nurses. In her words:

I feel very strongly that there's a lot of therapeutic skill that's involved – which is talked about in a dismissive way as basic nursing care. You know, bed-bathing, helping people to get dressed. I think it's the bringing together of those basic sorts of tasks which actually counts as something much more than that. It might include spending half an hour with someone, unpacking a lot of other issues and anxiety, worries, health issues or family. I think it's that rounded role which is difficult to articulate and difficult to defend when managers are asking for outputs. So I think there's a danger that nurses might lose that aspect of care with the move to substitution [re. doctors]. This is care that is, I think, valued by patients and it is what makes the work rewarding.

The respondent's words can be read as indicative of the way in which nurses can provide continuity to *individual* patients' lives. In this sense the words underline the view put forward in Chapter 3 that, for nurses, holistic care is about caring for the whole person. Continuity of care to specific groups was also a point of discussion. One general practitioner commented, 'as far as chronic diseases are concerned I honestly think that nurses probably do a better job.' She added:

I wouldn't have told you that five years ago, but the evidence now is that nurses are looking after the asthmatics better and looking after the diabetics and the hypertensives, providing they're routine. The routine stuff can be handled extremely well by practice nurses – immunization programmes are run by practice nurses. Practice nurses are better than doctors at doing routine audits – certainly carrying them out, and also in terms of planning what audit needs to be done.

One could read these words as indicative of how nurses might provide continuity of care to specialist areas of primary care. It is generally thought that nurses' career patterns tend towards work in specialist areas of care, unlike the general practitioner. One nurse respondent noted that 'even the GPs are becoming helpless saying "I can't help you with this child, but the nurse will see you" . . . so in *specialist* things like asthma and diabetes there's a shift in responsibility.' However, the emphasis in primary care nursing on specialism is changing; for example, in the training of nurse practitioners emphasis is placed on their generalist perspective (Barton *et al.* 1999). Practice nurses, too, have reported that while they may have particular responsibility for an area of specialist care, such as diabetes or care of women in the menopause, they are sometimes concerned that patients are seen by one nurse for, say, their menopause care and by another for, say, diabetes. As one respondent put it, 'I think there could be much greater continuity of care because, at the moment, particularly for the over 75s, you get put in touch with a different nurse for different bits of your anatomy.' Certainly, some nurses see for themselves a generalist role in much of their care. One nurse, a practice nurse, observed that 'doctors are at present at the centre of a health care system when they are basically trained for dealing with sickness.' This nurse was aware that promoting health has been a part of general practitioners' work since the inception of the Royal College of General Practitioners. Even so, she added: 'I don't necessarily agree with that. I think the nurses could be very much the centre – or we should allow the public to choose who their central person is going to be – it doesn't necessarily have to be the doctor.' And she noted 'how more people are opting to see a nurse in the practice rather than the doctor, especially where they have *immediate problems* with their chronic illness.' She made it clear that she was not referring to routine clinic visits, and concluded, 'I think things are changing. I think in some cases where nurses have been established for a while, the public, particularly in the cities, will go and get their help from the nurse.' She also added:

> As an experienced practice nurse, I should not be doing the routine urine testing and blood pressures but taking on more complex work. In the practice we have discussions about how we look after a patient with cardiac failure and how that is different from how the GP would. By that I mean what about their [patient's] skin and what about their diet? We as nurses would offer a different service from the GPs.

The practice nurse's words raise a number of important issues around development of the role and career of practice nurses. They also raise issues around continuity and fit between the service offered by medicine and the service offered by nursing. The majority of respondents emphasized the need for coordination and collaboration between the two professions, as has been discussed. For example, drawing on her experience as a district nurse, one study respondent noted that 'patients need to know who is going to be visiting them', adding:

> It's important to know, more or less, if people come to visit them, what is available in terms of information, services, and I think the more that's coordinated at a local level, the better you'll be able to deliver those sorts of things. You know, most of the patient satisfaction surveys when patients complain, it's about lack of planning, lack of feeling, sort of a disjointed approach to care . . . being put to bed at 7pm when they want to go to the party upstairs. You know, services which are not appropriate and individualized to what they the patients need. I think the more services are organized nearer the ground, the better that will happen. Which raises questions about the kind of overall planning, because the more you devolve, the more difficult it is to make sure that there is equity and that services are monitored and all those sorts of things which need to be done.

Her comments reflect a concern amongst community staff about the issue of timed appointments and the organization of community services required to implement these (McDonald 1996). She underlined the need for coordination and collaboration in the delivery of care using a personal anecdote:

> People are endlessly being assessed these days. My mother recently had a cataract in day care. The actual care was brilliant. Well, she was terribly happy about it, the actual operation. But they kept coming and asking questions – the same questions. And everyone was asking her about the same things – there was no sharing – no common plan – no common record. There's an awful lot of that around, not just in hospital, but in community care – for example the over 75 health check and endless questions. I think that's a violation . . .

This anecdote raises a key matter of current concern to policy makers and practitioners, both doctors and nurses. The need for better and coordinated information systems including shared patient records is pressing (Clark 1999). The technology is available. What is needed is work on setting up systems and then on the training of all categories of staff in order to make the system work. There will, however, be situations where technology is not enough. What is also needed is the will to coordinate care. One respondent was impressed with an innovative approach by nurses to the coordination of care in her region. She recounted a situation where:

> There were four nurses . . . they were cooperating in a different kind of role from usual. They were kind of brokers of care. Where there were problems where long-term care relationships go down, or whatever, they would be the first person the consultant phoned or the GP phoned. And they would go out and assess a problem and then get in touch with the relevant people. And they had the trust of the GPs. They were almost a health worker/social worker collapsed into one. They were really impressive.

Examples of innovative coordination of care led by nurses are increasing as indicated in Elliott's (1998) updated version of *Innovations in Primary Health Care Nursing*. Her review includes reference to care coordinated between the health care and other sectors including voluntary agencies, for example in the area of mental health and farming communities (Hughes 1996), between community development workers and the 'traditional public health approach' of health visiting in an estate seen as a pocket of deprivation in an otherwise relatively affluent area (Gilbert and Brett 1996). It includes examples of innovative joint initiative work across acute and primary care sectors as, for example, in the support of clients following laryngectomies (Feber 1996), facilitation of hospital discharge (Ware 1996) and continuing care at home (Buxton 1996). Certainly, there appears to be strong agreement that provision of continuity of care is a desirable 'outcome' for patients. How continuity of care is to be achieved will likely continue to tax all those involved in the delivery of care, not least nurses. Given the factors discussed above, there is also, to underline the point, a concern to identify more clearly the fit between medicine and nursing in providing continuity of care. It appears that there is agreement that nurses have an important role to play in coordinating this. This may be because, to reiterate one study respondent's expression, 'nurses do have a feel for something much broader in terms of what the delivery of humane care is about' – an observation which takes us to the next point of discussion.

Rethinking primary care

Innovation in primary care is about having new ideas about the delivery of care. In this sense, innovation refers to the demonstration of outcomes of care and clinically effective services (Elliott 1998). Some indication has been given in this chapter of the conditions necessary to promote such innovation. There remains, however, innovation at the conceptual level. Throughout this book, primary care has been conceived variously as the provision of a first-contact service within the UK, traditionally led by general practitioners, and as a service with the potential for the provision of care more widely defined. With recent changes in government and new policy drives, narrow conceptions of primary care are beginning to be challenged. For example, there is concern to incorporate a public health perspective (Welsh Office 1998b). Collaboration, as we have seen, is seen as critical to taking forward primary care (Department of Health 1998; Welsh Office 1998a) as are user-focused services (Welsh Office 1998c).

Study respondents' comments and observations made in 1996–97, by and large anticipated the mood for the policy changes prompted by the change in government in May 1997. One study respondent involved in nursing policy was critical of the lack of emphasis on prevention in primary care, and stressed the importance of the linkages between prevention, public health and working collaboratively. As noted in Chapter 4, she was concerned that 'a lot of primary care nurses . . . have lost a lot of their understanding of primary prevention' and emphasized the need for a public health perspective – a perspective which could be best fulfilled through 'multi-agency working'. She explained:

> Part of it is also recognizing that you don't do it on your own either, and that primary care is about recognizing the incredible importance of multi-agency working and that as a primary care practitioner you can achieve nothing unless you are cooperating with housing, social services, and social security and benefits – because if you're talking about prevention then that's what it's all about – prevention and not just about giving pills . . .

Her views on the necessity of prevention and a public health role were broadly shared by others within the study, although not all felt that nurses had lost their understanding for primary prevention entirely. One nurse ventured that 'where nurses manage chronic disease they do tend to embrace a preventative perspective'. Another felt that prevention of disease could not be taken for granted, and that indeed there is a place for nurses as well as general practitioners in being prepared to react to 'what comes through the door'. Indeed, nurses had much to offer. She elaborated:

> Well my thesis is – and you can pinch it! My thesis is that with the resurgence of infectious diseases and antibiotic resistance, nursing care – true nursing care – is going to come back into its own, and basically nurses have forgotten how to do it, and they are going to have to relearn. Yesterday I taught our child branch students about the major international issues in health care for children, and how they were war, the exploitation of child labour in the work force, the fate of girls, the missing women, and the resurgence of infectious diseases.

She continued:

> I said, in your lifetime as nurses you will encounter diseases that have only just emerged and diseases that have re-emerged which we thought had been conquered. I asked them if they knew what polio was and not one of them was able to tell me. Now I think that, for me, our education for nurses should not just be about the skills-based stuff – can you do a venepuncture or whatever – it is do you know enough of the basic sciences and how to apply them in order to be innovative and original so when you're confronted with something you know how to deal with it.

Her reference to antibiotic resistance and the need to be able to react innovatively was a point taken up by general practitioners in the study who were concerned that minor illnesses are not managed well by doctors, and who felt that nurses might provide a better outcome for patients through the use of alternative strategies to medication. The notion of alternative strategies was often invoked. A respondent involved in general practitioner training and education commented on the prescribing practices of colleagues, saying, 'one of the things we see with doctors during their training for general practice, and even at the end of it, is that they have a very limited repertoire of alternative strategies'. Another commented:

> I'm not all that convinced that general practitioners manage patients with minor self-limiting illness well; and in terms of minor self-limiting illness, nurses might manage it better because they are perhaps more reluctant to prescribe – or I should say seek a prescription. I think general practitioners over-prescribe in self-limiting conditions whereas there is very little evidence that patients benefit. They [GPs] hand it [medication] out like sweets.

He went on to suggest that:

> If nurses could actually offer something better than a prescription to somebody who comes in with, say, a sore throat – a consultation that

might involve something like reassurance, explanation of the natural history, what sorts of things will help and what won't work, what the patient can do – then the outcome could be better.

He added:

What is done during the consultation is important. It's not that difficult to diagnose a cold and it's not all that difficult to find out if there's more than a cold going on . . . so with a little more training a nurse . . . if the training is good . . . the outcome for patients could be better. Yes, I know there's the meningitis that comes in. That may fool any of us.

Another general practitioner recalled how a colleague had 'a nurse and a physio [physiotherapist] looking after patients with arthritis', emphasizing that no doctor was involved in the initiative. She commented that the nurse/physiotherapist team were 'actually reducing the prescriptions of analgesia', noting that, 'the nurse and the physio have to look at alternative ways of managing the disease other than prescribing'. From her perspective, nurses had developed a repertoire of care in the face of constraints imposed upon them as a profession, for example, constraints on prescribing. Her comments were made in the context of a discussion with the interviewer about what nurses stand to lose as their role expands. She was concerned that nurses might lose their capacity to 'work holistically'. She noted how 'Macmillan nurses work very holistically – and there's a danger that if they get into the therapeutic prescribing area that they will lose some of their skills looking for management strategies that involve things other then prescriptions.'

There are a number of ways of interpreting the general practitioners' comments on the idea of alternative strategies to prescribing. One is to say that general practitioners are concerned to provide a better service to patients, and see their comments as part of the wider debate about finding a fit between doctors' and nurses' work and responsibilities in order to provide better outcomes for patients. They, like nurses, recognize the value of rethinking approaches to primary care that draw for their justification on ideas about public health and collaboration. Another interpretation is that the general practitioners' comments reflect the process of shifting work from one group to another. The individuals who made the comments may not see it this way. However, as discussed in Chapter 3, analyses of similar shifts in work and responsibility suggest that once work becomes less challenging, or once basic ideas about work and established modes of working are challenged, then work is relinquished. In this case, we could read that an ability to cure has been challenged because of increasing resistance of bacteria to antibiotics, and that a subsequent duty to care – a duty which takes time and is difficult to market – is rejected. There is also an element of wanting to maintain professional boundaries by appealing to the ideas that have become part of the mythology of a profession – doctors cure and nurses care. Both professions, as we have seen in earlier chapters, engage in such boundary-marking.

The two readings of the general practitioners' words sit uneasily together. On the one hand, there is the possibility of collaboration, shared recognition of new challenges, and a sense of enterprise. The second reading suggests a negative form of professional allegiance. Inevitably, as we have suggested throughout, both readings have a bearing on the future.

It is possible to evaluate these readings in the light of a broader reading of the study findings which is that, despite major structural differences between the professions of nursing and medicine, despite different interpretations of ideas and core values, there is at least a point at which cultural convergence occurs between the various participants' comments and observations, whatever their professional or other allegiance. They are appealing to similar values, ideas and beliefs and the words they use are not so very different. This contrasts with what Wicks (1998) observed, at least in part of her study of nurses and doctors at work in the acute care sector in Sydney, Australia. She observed many examples of the dominance of the mechanistic and objectifying process of scientific medicine in the discourse and practice of the doctors. In one example, Wicks describes how, in a conversation between a doctor and a nurse, the words used by a doctor to describe a patient's 'condition' stood in stark contrast to the words used by the nurse 'to present . . . a human being who was suffering' (p. 163). From Wick's perspective, the conversation had no point at which the participants could meet.

In exploiting the potential for innovation in primary care, the engagement between the two major professions is critical. Nursing shares a commitment with medicine to care and to cure. It matters for patients that the fit between the two professions' contribution is coherent. Differences between the professions are positive if benefits for patients constitute the criterion for evaluating the professional contribution and not the privileging of one group over another. Medicine has had, and continues to maintain, a strong influence in shaping primary care. As discussed, nurses have a collective experience and approach which offers, in some respects, a critique of some aspects of current general practice medicine – a point made by general practitioners as well as nurses. It is important for nurses to overcome the uncertainties discussed in earlier chapters in order to engage with medical colleagues confidently and critically. This requires a shift in views about nursing at the highest level of society. As this chapter has shown, given the right preconditions the potential for innovation in primary health care is considerable.

6 Conclusion: cultural differences between medicine and nursing – implications for primary care

The chapters within this book have taken as their focus changes occurring on the boundary between medicine and nursing in the context of primary care. The boundary can be viewed as an ambiguous space – a culture of uncertainty – where traditional and taken-for-granted, professional identities are being challenged. As argued, uncertainty can either threaten or inspire the potential for innovation in primary care and this has been considered especially in relation to primary care nursing. Thus, much of the book's discussion has been concerned with identifying both the factors which threaten and the possibilities for exploiting the potential for innovation. In both cases, the emphasis has been on how seemingly contradictory ideas are interposed in order to give a sense of coherence and resolve to the work of doctors and, more particularly, to the work of nurses.

To conclude, I would like to comment on three key points of argument contained within the book. The first point is that doctors and nurses share culture. Second, there are important differences between the two professions, not least nursing's subordinate status in relation to medicine. Third, cultural differences between the two professions, especially differences in relation to status, will have implications for taking forward a primary care agenda where the emphasis is on cooperation, partnership and collaboration. This is because effective cooperation, partnership and collaboration between doctors and nurses depends on a nursing workforce which has confidence in its contribution to primary care. Confidence requires a sense of professional identity and purpose and, as argued in earlier chapters, this clearly needs to be balanced against current market imperatives for a needs-led, cost-effective service and flexible workforce rather than being undermined by them. The chapter draws to a close by suggesting a way forward in this respect.

Shared culture: ideas, values and beliefs held in common

In common with the rest of society, practitioners of primary care nursing and medicine draw on a broad range of ideas and shared values in order to justify their various practices. The ideas and values which influence contemporary life are divergent and seemingly contradictory thus, to reiterate, while doctors and nurses value compassion and the holistic dimension of their *engagement* with patients, they will at the same time value the sense of *detachment* associated with a spirit of critical enquiry, one which includes scientific enquiry. Doctors and nurses firmly believe in the centrality of the patient to all their endeavours, and a respect for the integrity of patients is paramount. At the same time, both have attended to the promotion of professional interests.

Medicine and nursing share not only a world of divergent and contradictory ideas but also a world in which ideas are creatively manipulated in order to support a particular point of view, to promote a political position or, possibly, to contain the power of competitors. For example, in the field of health care, the promotion of professional interests referred to by some as professional individualism has been challenged in recent years by a new version of individualism described by Frankford and Konrad (1998) as 'the world of managed care'. This, the authors suggest, is a version of individualism which has been created to avoid the 'collective power' of physicians, and it is one which has found expression in mechanisms to hold individual professionals accountable for their actions. Writing from a US perspective, the authors list these mechanisms as 'practice profiling, outcomes-based monitoring, economic credentialing, direct capitation of physicians within local markets, and the substitution of cheaper and more compliant forms of labor for the labor of physicians' (p. 140). The list will be familiar to UK health professionals who may read it as embodying the full collective force of a general management culture on the professions.

Frankford and Konrads' analysis forged in the US context is useful insofar as it signals the complexities of the political context of health care provision – a context where, from one perspective, an institution or practice is understood to be driven by cherished values held in common by its collective membership (for example, the duty of doctors and nurses to care and to cure; the duty of management to provide a cost-effective service and one that meets public demand); while from another perspective or at another point in time the same institution or practice is viewed as individualistic. From this perspective, caring and curing represent the drive for professional autonomy. Cost-effectiveness and public demand can be seen as the drive for power over professionals. To take another example, it is possible to read the recent UK White Papers on health care as espousing either collective or individualistic values, depending on one's point of view. The call for partnership and collaboration between professional groups and the desire to give patients' views greater emphasis can be read in two ways: firstly as a call for 'collective' action to improve the health of society; secondly, as an individualistic expression of 'managed care' the aim of which is to call into check the 'collective' power of professional or producer-led agendas for health. Some will choose to read it as either one or the other. It is perhaps more useful to recognize that, as is the case with most agendas for change, the White Papers constitute a dual, if seemingly contradictory, agenda in this respect.

Both the professions of medicine and nursing are familiar with a world of contradictory ideas around the justification of work and both engage in balancing professional interests against concern for the needs of others. Thus, there is correspondence between the two professions.

Cultural differences between medicine and nursing

There are of course differences and, as this book makes clear, difference is tied to variation in the interpretation of ideas and to inequalities in status between the two professions.

Differences in the interpretation and treatment of ideas, values and beliefs

While both nurses and doctors value ideas about care, holism and compassion, the ways in which these core values are interpreted and treated have differed significantly between medicine and nursing. To summarize one of the arguments developed here, the treatment of core ideas, values and beliefs depends on a number of factors linked to the differential histories and development of doctors and nurses working in primary care. For example, being a generalist in one's approach to practice is a key idea in general practice medicine and one which underpins the general practitioner's commitment to deal with a person seeking advice on a 'through the door' basis. Thus holism, care and compassion are shaped by a generalist perspective. They are also shaped by ideas about pathology, disease and epidemiology. Underpinning each of these ideas is the value placed on science.

In some contrast, specialist care is a feature of nurses' career pathways in primary care, so that ideas about holism and compassion take shape in relation to specific areas of care, for example in relation to chronic disease such as asthma and diabetes. Care related to women's reproductive lives, nurses' specialization in the care of older people and other areas have been identified. As discussed in Chapter 3, by virtue of its history, compassion, care and holism are shaped in nursing by a concern for knowing the individual as a whole person. Thus we may wish to distinguish between primary care medicine and nursing by saying that each discipline develops a significantly different relationship with patients or clients.

Changes are occurring in this respect. As nurses take on new roles, for example in consulting with patients about undifferentiated problems, then they too must be generalist in their approach, a point taken seriously by some who provide education and training for nurse practitioners, for example Barton *et al.* (1999). Also, the idea of science is taking greater prominence in primary care nursing as it is in nursing generally, and the evidence-based practice movement is now seen as critical. Specialist approaches to care are not totally outside the scope of general practice. General practitioners who may well have specialist qualifications themselves have a duty to address the epidemiology of need in relation to speciality services in general practice. At local level, 'audit systems, guidelines and purchasing plans need to be tested by how well they operate for a given specialty area across sectors in an illness episode or chronic care mode' (Boyd 1996: 23–4). Added to which, the new organization of primary care around primary care groups and their equivalents suggests that general practitioners might become more specialist in their approaches. Indeed, fears about a diminished generalist tradition in primary care have been voiced. Hunter, speaking at the NHS Confederation's 'All Our Tomorrows' conference in July 1998, is quoted as saying, 'We have to be attentive to the risk that we'll lose the generalist tradition in primary care' (Primary Care Network 1998: 1). It may become the case that cultural differences are not necessarily best assessed in relation to profession only, but rather in association with place and orientation of work.

Structural differences

Structurally, the relationship between medicine and nursing remains the same as it ever was. There is little substantial evidence to suggest that the historical relationship between the two professions is being seriously challenged. Some might suppose the new calls for collaboration and partnership in taking forward primary care will make a difference. However, as noted in Chapter 5, while some individual general practitioners are willing to collaborate – indeed to work in partnership with nurses and others – general practice medicine continues to be taken for granted as the leader in primary care, a point underlined throughout the book.

Some might also suppose that enterprise culture has set in motion the means by which the hierarchical relationship between medicine and nursing could be flattened. The argument rests in part on the view that market culture has, at least theoretically, made a difference to the health professional/client relationship so that once-passive users of health services are becoming more skilful in expressing their demands for the health service they want. Even so, as discussed in detail in Chapter 2, and reinforced throughout the book, the consumerist challenge to medicine's authority is still embryonic and there is little evidence to suggest that nurses face anything but an 'uphill struggle against the power of medicine' (Soothill 1998). As discussed in Chapter 3, recent proposals to flatten hierarchical ordering of health care professionals in schemes for the future tend to leave medicine out of the picture, at least in the UK context.

This said, the consumerist challenge while embryonic does exist. Writing from a US perspective, Frankford and Konrad (1998: 141) go so far as to suggest that 'users of professional labor increasingly define themselves as customers of medical education and are translating demands for the health service they want into prescriptive messages concerning the kinds of medical education they want "produced".' In Frankford and Konrad's words, lines of power are being reversed (p. 141). And while forces which serve towards equalizing the relationship between medicine and the public will not necessarily affect nursing's status in relation to medicine, the consumer challenge to medicine could pave the way for a division of health care labour based on ability to provide better outcomes for patients rather than on the privileging of one provider group over the other.

Implications for primary care

There are differences between medicine and nursing in the treatment and interpretation of ideas and there are structural differences. Of the two, it is perhaps the latter that is the most significant in relation to the future of primary care. Nursing has to date exerted some influence on policy makers but far less so than medicine. Calls for collaboration and partnership give nurses a degree of optimism in facing the future; however, efforts to check the power of professional groups look set to disadvantage nursing given its present status in relation to medicine. To reiterate, there is a danger that nursing's confidence will be eroded by this equivocal situation such that its potential to contribute effectively is threatened. Looking at the elements of the situation will throw some light upon the way forward.

The call for cooperation

In the National Health Service White Papers marking Labour's ascendancy in 1997 much has been made of the need for effective collaboration, partnership and cooperation in order to achieve a healthier society and to effect the reduction of health inequalities. Wilkinson (1996), who writes about ways of dealing with health inequalities, suggests that there are good arguments to support a collective, social and cohesive approach to the organization and delivery of health care. He suggests that such an approach helps to create a cohesive, moral community insofar as it draws on ideas about trust and taking the broader community interests into account. Viewed from this perspective, and as Wilkinson notes, it is an approach which finds expression in, for example, the British system for collecting blood for transfusion, a system where, in contrast to the US system, there is no commercial market in blood. Blood in the UK is given as a gift, freely and willingly with no expectation of immediate or necessary return (Titmuss 1970).

Wilkinson's argument does not rest entirely on the moral dimension of a socially cohesive approach. He refers to Putnam's (1995) concept of social capital. Putnam, a political scientist, describes the concept thus: 'Social capital, in short, refers to social connections and the attendant norms and trust', and 'features of social life – networks, norms and trust that enable participants to act together more effectively to pursue shared objectives' (1995: 664–5). Putnam continues, observing that, 'whether or not their [participants] shared goals are praiseworthy is, of course, entirely another matter'. He writes:

> To the extent that norms, networks, and trust link substantial sectors of the community and span underlying social cleavages – to the extent that the social capital is of a 'bridging' sort – then enhanced cooperation is likely to serve broader interests and to be widely welcomed. On the other hand, groups like the Michigan militia or youth gangs also embody a kind of social capital, for these networks and norms, too, enable members to cooperate more effectively, albeit to the detriment of the wider community.
>
> (p. 665)

Following Putnam in some respects, Wilkinson (1996) emphasizes how a collective, social and cohesive approach is a *pragmatic* solution (rather than a moral one) to the problem of effectiveness. His argument is that investment in social capital increases efficiency as well as effectiveness. This, he suggests, contrasts starkly with the economics of the 1980s and 1990s where, instead of a being a society where people share social bonds and common interests, we have acted as if we are competitors for jobs, for houses, space, seats on the bus, parking places, added to which are processes of social comparison – everything is constantly monitored. He suggests that economic systems such as this 'destroy a spirit of social cooperation' and 'may incur high additional costs as a result' (Wilkinson 1996: 221). The collective, social, cohesive approach does not, he stresses, mean that we are forced to choose between greater equity and economic growth. Rather it is a system incorporating both (see Williams *et al.* 1998: xx–xxi).

Maintaining a sense of professional identity – towards responsive professionalism

After exposure to almost two decades of competition within the National Health Service, there is something compelling about arguments for social

cooperation as a way forward for health care. The literature and respondents' comments within the NPCRDC study (as discussed in Chapter 5) echo
this view in their suggestions that if doctors and nurses (not forgetting
patients) work together collaboratively and in partnership, the likelihood of
better patient outcomes is greater than if they do not. As noted, contributors
to the literature and respondents alike fully recognize the difficulties, not
least a lack of confidence and absence of a clear sense of professional contribution. This latter point suggests that effective social cooperation is likely to
fail where confidence is lacking on the part of one of the collaborators or
partners. As argued throughout the book, a strong sense of professional
identity is a key to confidence. Thus, as mentioned in Chapter 4, it is not
enough to espouse consumerism and reject the idea of profession. Rather
there is a need to balance public confidence in health care with confidence
in one's professional contribution.

This said, 'professional autonomy', as conventionally conceived, empowers
the strongest at the expense of the weakest, often patients: a point made by
Stacey (1992) in her exposition of an agenda for the 'new professions'.
Stacey points to how the selfish aspects of profession get in the way of good
practice and she argues for a re-evaluation of profession, one which would
rebuild on the basis of the value of service and concern for the public good.
Her vision for the future of the profession of medicine is extended by
Hugman's (1991) concept of democratic professionalism as applied mainly
to nursing, physiotherapy and social work, whereby the creation of partnerships with clients and a concern for enabling clients' direct participation in
decision making at the level of service delivery offers the possibility of a
sense of profession which is not only responsive to the needs of society, but
also displays a reflexive awareness of issues of power and of status (see also
Chapman *et al.* 1994). As noted in Chapter 4, Davies (1995, 1996a) does not
entirely reject the possibility of a new model of profession for nursing, one
which would involve a 'practitioner' who is engaged, embodied and creating
an active problem-solving environment' (Davies 1995: 185) as well as being
interdependent (p. 149).

Echoing some aspects of the above analyses, Frankford and Konrad (1998)
argue, 'the medical profession must recognize that traditional individualistic
professional autonomy is no longer a viable path'. Writing from a US perspective about medical education, Frankford and Konrad assert, 'in the face
of market imperatives, professionalism can survive only if it is reformu-
lated', and they continue by saying that professionalism 'must be more
explicitly responsive to society, but responsive in a manner quite different
from that proposed by current attempts merely to accommodate medical
education to market demands' (p. 144). They continue, 'As sympathetic lay
observers, we [the authors] may be in a position to identify the general
nature of what should be done . . . Members of the medical profession, who
are the participants in the task of caregiving are the best persons to delineate
the intricacy of the task' (p. 144).

While the general direction of the latter proposal is fine, there are one or two problems. The first is that the authors may be too hasty in their assessment of the relevance of a patient point of view to 'the intricacies of the task'. Given that the intricacies of the task normally centre on the professional/patient relationship, it is highly likely that the latter point of view will be important. Second, depending on what the authors mean by general, it may be the case that a professional point of view is important in sketching the general nature of what should be done. For example, should not health professionals concern themselves with health care at the level of policy?

There is clearly a strong imperative for both medicine and nursing to increase their responsiveness to society in relation to everyday practice and at the level of policy, both operational and strategic. The professions must also, as Frankford and Konrad discuss in detail, be aware that users of health services are increasingly defining themselves as 'customers of medical education' (and, by extension, nursing education), a point which has echoes in recent comments from the Committee of Vice Chancellors and Principals, as discussed in Chapter 5. Similarly, it would appear to follow that users of health services would be interested in health services research and development.

From a nursing perspective, it is important that nurses strike a balance between developing responsiveness to the public (both potential users of care and patients) on the one hand, and developing and promoting their expertise and professional contribution on the other. A critical point in the present argument is that it is important not to lose sight of the fact that a more responsive professionalism depends in part on practitioners who are confident about their professional contribution and who are able to promote it. They must also be willing to listen and to negotiate.

On the first point, ideas about holism, compassion and caring are difficult to promote and market, as has been identified, and how these ideas are promoted is critical to a recognition of the differential contributions of medicine and nursing to primary care. For example, holism promoted as relational and person-centred may be rejected in favour of holism promoted as scientific and pathology orientated. This is in part a function of the value placed on science. In part it relates to a particular view of what constitutes evidence, with the randomized controlled trial as the benchmark in producing evidence. In some instances nurses may wish to promote the latter. However, rejection of holism promoted as relational is also, in part, due to a lack of confidence and creativity in finding ways to measure the value of ideas which are hard to define and which have been, and may remain, central not only to nursing but also, importantly, to the health of individual patients and to a healthy society. Nurses may wish to promote research which aims to extend the boundaries of what counts as evidence.

Research will assist in the promotion of nursing contributions to primary care and it should be accomplished in conjunction with a responsiveness to expressed public needs. For example, in the UK, concern to increase flexibility of access to primary health care is driving new schemes such as NHS Direct and the proposed new venues for primary care, including drop-in centres where an appointment is not necessary. In both examples of flexible access to primary care, nurses are likely to be the first point of contact for advice. There remain needs as yet unmet by the system, particularly the needs of those who are not registered with a general practitioner, for example travellers and the homeless. Nurses may wish to take the lead in progressing collaborative ventures to extend the boundaries of primary care in order to provide a more inclusive service.

In the system as it currently stands, there is an opportunity to test 'responsive professionalism' in the newly formed primary care groups, local health groups and their equivalents. Responsiveness, democracy and new professionalism each encompass the imperative to take into account all stakeholder views. There is a danger that in the enthusiasm to get the work done, some views in these critical decision-making groups may be overlooked. General practitioners are in the majority, and there is a real danger that the views of other stakeholders could be subordinated. They may not be heard at all because lack of confidence prevents them from being expressed. This could be the case for those representing the public point of view. It could be the case for those representing nursing who have the task of ensuring that nursing views on health issues are heard, taken seriously, negotiated if necessary and acted upon – not an easy feat in a formal meeting where the majority are members of a profession which traditionally has viewed itself as superior to nursing.

The need to ensure that nursing views are heard and taken seriously is urgent. As previously noted, nurses' collective experience provides the basis for a positive critique of accepted knowledge and practice in some areas of primary care medicine. It is important that the critique is heard. For its part, the profession of nursing must embrace the will to work collaboratively. As indicated in Chapter 5, cooperation, partnership and collaboration is very likely the best chance that nurses have for taking forward a primary care that provides better outcomes for patients. Paradoxically it may be that in working to establish a clear, strong sense of professional identity, contribution and purpose, nurses will feel able to move beyond the point of retreat into the protection of 'profession' or, as Salmon (1999: 173) puts it 'a nursing centric . . . professional purism', to the centre-stage of cooperative health care provision – the place where the action is and where nurses have much to contribute. Nursing has always played a critical role in primary care. A broader collaborative vision of that role is the way forward.

Bibliography

Abbott, A. (1988) *The System of the Professions*. Chicago: University of Chicago Press.

Abercrombie, N. (1994) Authority and consumer society, in R. Keat, N. Whiteley and N. Abercrombie (eds) *The Authority of the Consumer*. London: Routledge.

Adorian, D., Silverberg, D.S., Tomer, D. and Womasher, Z. (1990) Group discussions with the health care team: a method of improving care of hypertension in general practice, *Journal of Human Hypertension*, 4(3): 265–8.

Alford, R. (1975) *Health Care Politics*. Chicago: Chicago University Press.

Annandale, E. (1996) Working on the front line: risk culture and nursing in the new NHS, *Sociological Review*, 44(3): 416–51.

Anonymous (1996) Are nurse practitioners merely substitute doctors? *Professional Nurse*, 11(5): 325–8.

Armstrong, D. (1979) The Emancipation of biographical medicine, *Social Science and Medicine*, 13: 1–3.

Armstrong, D. (1995) The rise of surveillance medicine, *Sociology of Health and Illness*, 17(3): 405–17.

Ashby, M., Kissane, D., Beadle, G. and Roger, A. (1996) Psychosocial support, treatment of metastic disease and palliative care, *Medical Journal of Australia*, 164(1): 43–9.

Ashton, J. and Seymour, H. (1988) *The New Public Health*. Milton Keynes: Open University Press.

Atkin, K. and Lunt, N. (1993) *Nurses Count. A National Census of Practice Nurses*. York: Social Policy Research Unit, University of York.

Atkin, K. and Lunt, N. (1996) Negotiating the role of the practice nurse in general practice, *Journal of Advanced Nursing*, 24: 498–505.

Atkins, S. and Williams, A. (1994) Registered nurses' experiences of mentoring undergraduate nursing students, *Journal of Advanced Nursing*, 21: 1006–166.

Bailey, J. (1996) Using nursing theory to introduce change in practice, *Nursing Standard*, 10(51): 40–3.

Barton, T.D., Thome, R. and Hoptroff, M. (1999) The nurse practitioner: redefining occupational boundaries, *International Journal of Nursing Studies*, 36: 57–63.

Bates, B. (1970) Doctor and nurse: changing roles and relations, *New England Journal of Medicine*, 283(3): 129–34.

Beck, U. (1992) *Risk Society: Towards a New Modernity*. London: Sage.

Beddow, T., Clark, J., Delahunty, A., Gibbons, B. and Tudor Hart, J. (1998) *Locality*

Commissioning and Salaried Primary Care. Swansea: Swansea and District Socialist Health Association.

Bentley, H. (1991) Back to the future, *Nursing Times*, 87(24): 29–30.

Bloor, M. and McIntosh, J. (1990) Surveillance and concealment: a comparison of techniques of client resistance in therapeutic communities and health visiting, in S. Cunningham Burley and N. McKeganey, *Readings in Medical Sociology*. London: Routledge.

Bolman, W.M. (1995) The place of behavioural science in medical education and practice, *Academic Medicine*, 70(10): 873–8.

Bond, S., Cartilidge, A.M., Gregson, B.A., Philips, P.R., Bolam, F. and Gill, K.M. (1985) *A Study of Inter-professional Collaboration in Primary Health Care Organisations*, Report No. 27, Vol. 2. Newcastle-upon-Tyne: Health Care Research Unit, University of Newcastle-upon-Tyne.

Bond, S., Cunningham, B., Sargeant, S. *et al.* (1998) *Evaluation of Nurse Practitioners in General Practice in Northumberland*, Report No. 84. Newcastle-upon-Tyne: Centre for Health Services Research, University of Newcastle-upon-Tyne.

Bowles, A. (1992) What is a nurse practitioner? *Practice Nurse*, 4(8): 452–3.

Bowling, A. (1996) The role of practice nurses in the UK – from doctor's assistant to collaborative practitioner, in A. Bowling and B. Stilwell (eds) *The Nurse in Family Practice: Practice Nurses and Nurse Practitioners in Primary Health Care*. London: Baillière Tindall.

Bowling, A. and Stilwell, B. (1988) *The Nurse in Family Practice*. London: Scutari.

Bowling, A. and Stilwell, B. (1996) *The Nurse in Family Practice: Practice Nurses and Nurse Practitioners in Primary Health Care*. London: Baillière Tindall.

Boyd, R. (1996) Challenges to a primary care-led NHS: a medical specialist's view, in *What is the Future for a Primary Care Led NHS?* Manchester: NPCRDC.

Bradshaw, A. (1996) Nursing and medicine: co-operation or conflict? *British Medical Journal*, 311: 304–5.

Broadbent, J. and Laughlin, R. (1997) Contractual changes in schools and general practices: professional resistance and the role of absorption and absorbing groups, in R. Flynn and G. Williams (eds) *Contracting for Health*. Oxford: Oxford University Press.

Brooks, F. and Phillips, D. (1996) Do women want women health workers? Women's views of the primary health care service, *Journal of Advanced Nursing*, 23: 1207–11.

Bunker, J. (1994) Can professionalism survive in the marketplace? *British Medical Journal*, 308: 1179–80.

Butterworth, T. (1999) Nursing a grievance, *Times Higher Education Supplement*, 22 January.

Buxton, V. (1996) Freedom of choice, *Nursing Times*, 92(43): 57–9.

Calnan, M. and Williams, S. (1992) Images of scientific medicine, *Sociology of Health and Illness*, 14: 233–55.

Carlisle, R.D. and Johnstone, S. (1996) Factors influencing the response to advertisements for general practice vacancies, *British Medical Journal*, 313: 468–71.

Cassidy, J. (1996) Job swap, *Nursing Times*, 92(28): 20.

Cater, L. and Hawthorn, P. (1996) A survey of practice nurses in the UK – their extended roles, in A. Bowling and B. Stilwell (eds) *The Nurse in Family Practice: Practice Nurses and Nurse Practitioners in Primary Health Care*. London: Baillière Tindall.

Chapman, T., Hugman, R. and Williams, A. (1994) Effectiveness of interpersonal relationships: a case illustration of joint working, in L. Mackay, K. Soothill and C. Webb (eds) *Interprofessional Relations in Health Care*. London: Edward Arnold.

Choi, M. (1995) The menopausal transition: change, loss and adaptation, *Holistic Nursing Practice*, 9(3): 53–62.

Clark, J. (1999) Personal communication, 21 July.

Clement, J., Kinnersley, P., Howard, E. *et al.* (1999) *A randomised controlled trial of nurse practitioner versus general practice care for patients with acute illnesses in primary care: executive summary*. Cardiff: Department of General Practice, Llanedeyrn Health Centre.

Cornwell, J. (1986) *Hard Earned Lives*. London: Tavistock.

Cowley, S. (1995) In health visiting a routine visit is one that has passed, *Journal of Advanced Nursing*, 22(2): 276–84.

Cox, D. (1991) Health service management – a sociological view: Griffiths and the non-negotiated order of the hospital, in J. Gabe, M. Calnan and M. Bury (eds) *The Sociology of the Health Service*. London: Routledge.

Crompton, R. (1990) Professions in the current context, *Work, Employment and Society*, Special Issue: 147–66.

Crompton, R. (1996) Paid employment and the changing system of gender relations, *Sociology*, 30(3): 427–45.

Davies, C. (ed.) (1980) *Rewriting Nursing History*. London: Croom Helm.

Davies, C. (1984) General practitioners and the pull of prevention, *Sociology of Health and Illness*, 6(3): 267–89.

Davies, C. (1995) *Gender and the Professional Predicament in Nursing*. Buckingham: Open University Press.

Davies, C. (1996a) The sociology of the professions and the profession of gender, *Sociology*, 30(4): 661–78.

Davies, C. (1996b) A new vision of professionalism, *Nursing Times*, 92(46): 54–6.

Deeks, J., Glanville, J. and Sheldon, T. (1996) *Undertaking Systematic Reviews of Research on Effectiveness*. York: Centre for Reviews and Dissemination, University of York.

Denner, S. (1995) Extending professional practice: benefits and pitfalls, *Nursing Times*, 91(14): 27–9.

Department of Health (1989) *Working for Patients*, Cm 555. London: HMSO.

Department of Health (1991a) GPs Workload Survey 1989–90, vol. 1. Economic Research Unit. GP Manpower in England and Wales Quarterly Bulletin. BMA 7,3.

Department of Health (1991b) *The Health of the Nation*, Cm 1523. London: HMSO.

Department of Health (1992) *The Health of the Nation: A Strategy for Health in England*, Cm 1986. London: HMSO.

Department of Health (1993a) *Nursing in Primary Health Care: New World, New Opportunities*. Leeds: National Health Service Executive.

Department of Health (1993b) *Report of the Taskforce on the Strategy for Research in Nursing, Midwifery and Health Visiting*. Leeds: National Health Service Executive.

Department of Health (1996a) *Choice and Opportunity: Primary Care the Future*. London: The Stationery Office Limited.

Department of Health (1996b) *Primary Care: Delivering the Future*. London: The Stationery Office Limited.

Department of Health (1998) *The New NHS: Modern Dependable*, White Paper. London: The Stationery Office Limited.

Department of Health and Social Security (1983) *NHS Management Enquiry* (Griffiths Report). London: HMSO.

Department of Health and Social Security (1986a) *Neighbourhood Nursing. A Focus for Care* (Cumberlege Report), Report of the Community Nursing Review. London: HMSO.

Department of Health and Social Security (1986b) *Primary Health Care. An Agenda for Discussion*. London: HMSO.

Department of Health and Social Security (1987) *Promoting Better Health: The Government's Programme for Improving Primary Health Care*. London: HMSO.

Deveraux, M. (1991) *Nurse Practitioners in North America*. London: Kings Fund.

Ditzenberger, G., Collins, S. and Banta-Wright, S. (1995) Combining the roles of clinical nurse specialist and neonatal nurse practitioner: the experience in one academic tertiary care setting, *Journal of Perinatal and Neonatal Nursing*, 9(3): 45–52.

Dontje, K.J., Sparks, B.T. and Given, B.A. (1996) Establishing a collaborative practice in a comprehensive breast clinic, *Clinical Nurse Specialist*, 10(2): 95–101.

Dowling, S., Barrett, S. and West, R. (1995) With nurse practitioners, who needs house officers? *British Medical Journal*, 311: 274–5.

Elliott, M. (1998) *Innovations in Primary Health Care Nursing*, 2nd edn. Edinburgh: CDNA.

Elston, M.A. (1991) The politics of professional power: medicine in a changing health service, in J. Gabe, M. Calnan and M. Bury (eds) *The Sociology of the Health Service*. London: Routledge.

Fagermoen, M.S. (1997) Professional identity: values embedded in meaningful nursing practice, *Journal of Advanced Nursing*, 25: 434–41.

Feber, P. (1996) *Nursing Times*, 92(48): 50–1.

Feldman, J., Ventura, M.R. and Crosby, F. (1987) Studies of nurse practitioner effectiveness, *Nursing Research*, 36(5): 303–8.

Finch, J. (1984) 'It's great to have someone to talk to': the ethics and politics of interviewing women, in C. Bell and H. Roberts (eds) *Social Researching*. London: Routledge & Kegan Paul.

Flynn, R. and Williams, G. (1997) *Contracting for Health*. Oxford: Oxford University Press.

Flynn, R., Williams, G. and Pickard, S. (1996) *Markets and Networks: Contracting in Community Health Services*. Buckingham: Open University Press.

Foucault, M. (1973) *The Birth of the Clinic: An Archaeology of Medical Perception*. London: Tavistock.

Foucault, M. (1977) *Discipline and Punishment*. London: Allen Lane.

Foucault, M. (1980) The eye of power, in C. Gordon (ed.) *Power/Knowledge*. Brighton: Harvester Press.

Fournier, V. (1997) Boundary work and the making of the professions. Paper presented at the conference 'Professionalism, Boundaries and the Workplace', University of Derby, 1 February.

Fox, N. (1993) *Postmodernism, Sociology and Health*. Buckingham: Open University Press.

Fox, R.C. (1994) *Experiment Perilous*. Philadelphia, CA: University of Pennsylvania Press.

Fox, R.C. and Swazey, J.P. (1974) *The Courage to Fail: A Social View of Organ Transplants and Dialysis*. Chicago: University of Chicago Press.

Frankford, D.M. and Konrad, T.R. (1998) Responsive medical professionalism: integrating education, practice and community in a market-driven era, *Academic Medicine*, 73(2): 138–45.

Freeman, G. and Richards, S. (1993) Is personal continuity of care compatible with free choice of doctor? Patients' views on seeing the same doctor, *British Journal of General Practice*, 43: 493–7.

Gabe, J. and Calnan, M. (1989) The limits of medicine: women's perception of medical technology, *Social Science and Medicine*, 28(3): 223–31.

Gabe, J., Gustafasson, U. and Bury, M. (1991) Newspaper cover of tranquilliser dependence, *Sociology of Health and Illness*, 13: 332–51.

Garbett, R. (1996a) The growth of nurse-led care, *Nursing Times*, 92(1): 29.

Garbett, R. (1996b) Second sight care, *Nursing Times*, 92(29): 42–3.

General Medical Services (1995) *GMS Statistics*. London: British Medical Association.

General Medical Services Committee (1986) *Report to the Special Conference of Representatives of Local Medical Committees*. London: British Medical Association.

General Medical Services Committee (1996a) *Defining Core Services in General Practice – Reclaiming Professional Control*. London: British Medical Association.

General Medical Services Committee (1996b) *Medical Workforce Task Group Report*. London: British Medical Association.

Gibbings, S. (1995) Dependency, skill mix and grade mix and their effects on health visiting practice, *Journal of Clinical Nursing*, 4: 43–7.

Gibbs, I., McCaughan, D. and Griffiths, M. (1991) Skill mix in nursing: a selective review of the literature, *Journal of Advanced Nursing*, 16: 242–9.

Giddens, A. (1973) *The Class Structure of Advanced Societies*. London: Hutchinson.

Giddens, A. (1986) *Sociology: A Brief but Critical Introduction*, 2nd edn. London: Macmillan.

Gilbert, A. and Brett, S. (1996) A public health nursing post: the tools for getting started, *Nursing Times*, 92(16): 33–5.

Gillman, J., Gable-Rodriguez, J., Sutherland, S. and Whitacre, R. (1996) Pastoral care in a critical setting, *Critical Care Nursing Quarterly*, 19(1): 10–20.

Glaser, P. and Slater, M. (1987) *Unequal Colleagues: The Entrance of Women into the Professions 1890–1940*. New Brunswick: Rutgers University Press.

Graham, R. and West, J. (1996) The role of the rheumatology nurse practitioner in primary care: an experiment in the further education of the practice nurse, *British Journal of Rheumatology*, 35: 581–8.

Green, B., Jones, M., Hughes, D. and Williams, A. (1998) *Primary Care Information for Action*. Swansea: School of Health Science, University of Wales.

Hall, M., McCormack, P., Arthurs, N. and Freely, J. (1995) The spontaneous reporting of adverse drug reactions by nurses, *British Journal of Clinical Pharmacology*, 40(2): 173–5.

Hammersley, M. and Atkinson, P. (1995) *Ethnography: Principles in Practice*, 2nd edn. London: Routledge.

Hancock, C. (1997) Stand by for supernurse, *Health Services Journal*, 9 January: 17.

Harrison, S. and Pollitt, C. (1995) *Controlling Health Professionals: The Future of Work and Organisation in the National Health Service*. Buckingham: Open University Press.

Health Policy and Economic Research Unit (1996) *Quarterly Bulletin*, vol. 11, no. 3. London: British Medical Association.

Health Policy and Economic Research Unit (1998) *Career Intentions of 1st Year Senior House Officers*. British Medical Association Cohort Study of 1995 Medical Graduates, Third Report. London: British Medical Association.

Health Promotion Wales (1998) *A Community Approach to Primary Care: Report of a Conference*. Cardiff: Health Promotion Wales.

Health Services Management Unit (1996) *The Future Healthcare Workforce*, Steering Group Report. Manchester: HSMU, University of Manchester.

Healy, P. (1996) 'Scope' brings liberation, *Nursing Standard*, 10(31): 14.

Heath, I. (1995) *The Mystery of General Practice*. London: Nuffield Provincial Hospitals Trust.

Hiscock, J. and Pearson, M. (1996) Professional costs and invisible value in the community nursing market, *Journal of Interprofessional Care*, 10(1): 23–31.

Hoffman, E. and Redman, J. (1995) Physician assistants and nurse practitioners in Louisiana, *Journal of Louisiana State Medical Society*, 147(6): 267–79.

Holland, W.W. (ed.) (1983) *Evaluation of Health Care*. Oxford: Oxford University Press.

Hopkins, A., Solomon, J. and Abelson, J. (1996) Shifting boundaries in professional care, *Journal of the Royal Society of Medicine*, 89(7): 364–71.

Howard, S. (1999) Nurse education – scapegoating and gender stereotyping, *AUT Woman*, 46, Spring.

Hughes, D. (1988) When nurse knows best: some aspects of nurse/doctor relationships in a casualty department, *Sociology of Health and Illness*, 10(1): 1–22.

Hughes, H. (1996) Preventing suicide among isolated farmers, *Community Nurse*, 2(6): 12–13.

Hugman, R. (1991) *Power in the Caring Professions*. London: Macmillan.

Hurst, R. (1996) Looking beyond the presenting problem, *Australian Family Physician*, 25(11): 1693–7.

Illich, I. (1975) *Medical Nemisis: The Expropriation of Health*. London: Calder & Boyers.

Irvine, D. (1993) General practice in the 1990s: a personal view on future developments, *British Journal of General Practice*, 43: 121–5.

Jenkins Clarke, S., Carr-Hill, R. and Dixon, P. (1998) Teams and seams: skill mix in primary care, *Journal of Advanced Nursing*, 28(5): 1120–6.

Johnstone, T. (1971) *Professions and Power*. London: Macmillan.

Jones, R.V.H. (1992) Teamwork in primary care: how much do we know about it? *Journal of Interprofessional Care*, 6: 25–9.

Jordan, S. (1994) Nurse practitioners, learning from the USA experience: a review of the literature, *Health and Social Care in the Community*, 2(3): 173–86.

Karpf, A. (1988) *Doctoring the Media: The Reporting of Health and Medicine*. London: Routledge.

Kaufman, G. (1996) Nurse practitioners in general practice: an expanded role, *Nursing Standard*, 11(8): 44–7.

Keat, R. (1991) Consumer sovereignty and the integrity of practices, in R. Keat and N. Abercrombie (eds) *Enterprise Culture*. London: Routledge.

Keat, R. and Abercrombie, N. (1991) *Enterprise Culture*. London: Routledge.

Kelly, A. (1996) The concept of the specialist community nurse, *Journal of Advanced Nursing*, 24: 42–52.

Kinnersley, P. *et al.* (2000) Randomised controlled trial of nurse practitioner versus general practitioner care for patients requesting 'same day' consultations in primary care, *British Medical Journal*, 320: 1043–8.

Kocurek, K. (1996) Primary care of the HIV patient: standard practice and new developments in the era of managed care, *Medical Clinics of North America*, 80(2): 375–410.

Lambert, T., Goldacre, M., Edwards, C. and Parkhouse, J. (1996) Career preferences of doctors who qualified in the United Kingdom in 1993 compared with those of doctors qualifying in 1974, 1977, 1980, and 1983, *British Medical Journal*, 31: 19–24.

Larkin, G. (1983) *Occupational Monopoly and Modern Medicine*. London: Tavistock.

Lawson, N. (1999) *The Observer*, 17 January.

Lenehan, C. and Watts, A. (1994) Nurse practitioners in primary care: here to stay, *British Journal of General Practice*, July: 291–2.

LeVine, R.A. (1986) Properties of culture: an ethnographic view, in R.A. Schweder and R.A. LeVine (eds) *Culture Theory: Essays on Mind, Theory and Emotion*. Cambridge: Cambridge University Press.

Lewis, J. (1996) Primary health care for homeless people in A and E, *Professional Nurse*, 12(1): 13–18.

Lewis, J. (1997) *Independent Contractors. GPs and the GP Contract in the Post-War Period. Debates in Primary Care.* Manchester: National Primary Care Research and Development Centre.

Lilley, R. (1999) Nursing shortage and NHS decline. Letter to *The Times*, 12 September.

Long, S. (1996) Primary health care team workforce: team members' perspectives, *Journal of Advanced Nursing*, 23: 935–41.

Louria, D. (1995) The future of health care and the medical profession in the United States, *New Jersey Medicine*, 92(10): 667–9.

Love, C. (1995) Orthopaedic nursing: a study of its specialist status, *Nursing Standard*, 9(44): 36–40.

Lupton, D. (1995) *Medicine as Culture: Illness, Disease and the Body in Western Societies.* London: Sage.

Mackay, L. (1993) *Conflicts in Care: Medicine and Nursing.* London: Chapman & Hall.

Mackie, C. (1996) Nurse-led clinics: nurse practitioners managing anticoagulant clinics, *Nursing Times*, 92(1): 25–6.

Mahoney, D.F. (1988) An economic analysis of the nurse practitioner, *Nurse Practitioner*, 13(3): 44–52.

Marcus, J. (1997) Doctors take a lesson in caring, *Times Higher Education Supplement*, 14 March.

Marsh, G. (1967) Group practice nurse: an analysis and comment on six months' work, *British Medical Journal*, 1: 489–91.

Marsh, G. and Dawes, M.L. (1995) Establishing a minor illness clinic in a busy general practice, *British Medical Journal*, 310(6982): 778–80.

Martin, E. (1999) Letter to *The Guardian*, 19 February.

Mathieson, A. (1996) Anger at 'mini-doctor' jibe, *Nursing Standard*, 4(10): 15.

May, C. (1991) Affective neutrality and involvement in nurse–patient relationships: perceptions of appropriate behaviour among nurses in acute medical and surgical wards, *Journal of Advanced Nursing*, 16: 552–8.

May, C. (1992) Nursing work, nurses' knowledge, and the subjectification of the patient, *Sociology of Health and Illness*, 14(4): 472–87.

Maynard, A. and Bloor, K. (1993) Cost effective prescribing of pharmaceuticals: the search for the holy grail? in A. Maynard and F. Drummond (eds) *Purchasing and Providing Cost Effective Health Care.* Edinburgh: Churchill Livingstone.

McDonald, P. (1996) Can timed appointments for community staff improve care? *Nursing Times*, 92(18): 35–7.

McKinlay, J. and Archer, J. (1985) Towards the proletarianization of professions, *International Journal of Health Services*, 15: 161–95.

McKinlay, J.B. and Stoeckle, J.D. (1988) Corporatization and the social transformation of doctoring, *International Journal of Health Studies*, 18(2): 191–205.

Meyer, J. and Spilsbury, K. (1998) *Defining the Nursing Contribution.* London: St Bartholomew School of Nursing and Midwifery, City University.

Mottram, E. (1968) Extended use of nursing services in general practice, *Nursing Mirror*, 126: 20–4.

Murray, J. (1967) Fifteen years in general practice, *Journal of the Royal College of General Practitioners*, 13: 367.

Myerson, S. (1992) Workload in general practice under the new contract, *Health Service Management*, 88: 25–26.

National Health Service Executive (1997a) *R&D in Primary Care* (Mant Report). London: Department of Health.
National Health Service Executive (1997b) *Salaried Doctor's Scheme*, FHSL(97)46. Leeds: NHS Executive.
National Health Service Executive (1998) *The New NHS Modern and Dependable. Developing Primary Care Groups*. Health Service Circular HSC 1998/139. Leeds: NHS Executive.
National Health Service Management Executive (1993) *New World, New Opportunities – Nursing in Primary Care*. London: NHSME.
Nettleton, S. (1995) *The Sociology of Health and Illness*. Oxford: Polity Press.
Neufer, L. (1994) The role of the community nurse in environmental health, *Public Health Nursing*, 11(3): 155–62.
Nightingale, F. (1952) *Notes on Nursing*. London: Gerald Duckworth.
Oakely, A. (1980) Interviewing women: a contradiction in terms, in H. Roberts (ed.) *Doing Feminist Research*. London: Routledge & Kegan Paul.
Office of Technology Assessment (1986) *Nurse Practitioners, Physician Assistants, and Certified Nurse-midwives: A Policy Analysis*, Health Technology Case Study 37. Washington DC: Office of Technology Assessment.
Okely, J. (1996) *Own or Other Culture*. London: Routledge.
Oswald, N. (1992) The history and development of the referral system, in M. Roland and A. Coulter (eds) *Hospital Referrals*. Oxford: Oxford University Press.
Øvretveit, J. (1998) *Evaluating Health Interventions*. Buckingham: Open University Press.
Owen, M. and Holmes, C. (1993) 'Holism' in the Discourse of Nursing, *Journal of Advanced Nursing*, 18: 1688–95.
Paxton, F., Porter, M. and Heaney, D. (1996) Evaluating the workload of practice nurses: a study, *Nursing Standard*, 10(21): 33–8.
Pearson, R. (1985) Asthma clinic success story, *Pulse*, 8 June: 59.
Peckham, S. and Winters, M. (1996) Unequal approach, *Nursing Times*, 92(12): 31–5.
Pedersen, L.L. and Leese, B. (1997) What will a primary care led NHS mean for GP workload? The problem of the lack of an evidence base, *British Medical Journal*, 314: 1337–41.
Peiro, J., Gonzalez-Roma, V. and Ramos, J. (1992) The influence of work team climate on role, stress, tension, satisfaction and leadership perceptions, *European Review of Applied Psychology*, 42(1): 49–56.
Peter, A. (1993) Practice nursing in Glasgow after the new general practitioner contract, *British Journal of General Practice*, 43: 97–100.
Pickersgill, F. (1995) A natural extension, *Nursing Times*, 91(30): 24–7.
Porter, S. (1995) *Nursing's Relationship with Medicine*. Aldershot: Avebury.
Poulton, B.C. and West, M. (1993) Effective multidisciplinary teamwork in primary health care, *Journal of Advanced Nursing*, 18: 918–25.
Primary Care Network (1998) PCGs are off and rolling, *Primary Care Network: an Information Resource Service*, 2(2): 1.
Putnam, R.D. (1995) Tuning in, tuning out: the strangest disappearance of social capital in America, *Political Science and Politics*, December: 664–83.
Quinney, D. and Pearson, M. (1996) Different Worlds, Missed Opportunities? Primary Health Care Nursing in a North Western Health District. Report 96/24 Working paper 4. Liverpool, The Health and Community Care Research Unit.
Rafferty, A.M. (1997) Does nursing have a future? *Image Journal of Nursing Scholarship*, 29(2): 111–15.
Rafferty, A.M. (1999) Practice made perfect, *Guardian Higher*, 26 January.

Rashid, A., Watts, A. and Lenehan, C. (1996) Skill mix in primary care: sharing clinical workload and understanding professional roles, editorial, *British Journal of General Practice*, November: 639–40.

Rees, M. and Kinnersley, P. (1996) Nurse-led management of minor illness in a GP surgery, *Nursing Times*, 92(6): 32–3.

Reveley, S. (1998) The role of the triage nurse practitioner in general medical practice: an analysis of the role, *Journal of Advanced Nursing*, 28(3): 584–91.

Richardson, G. and Maynard, A. (1995) *Fewer Doctors? More Nurses? A Review of the Knowledge Base of Nurse–Doctor Substitution*. Discussion Paper 135. York: Centre for Health Economics, University of York.

Richardson, S. (1997) Integrated approach is a success, *General Practitioner*, January: 33.

Ridsdale, L. (1993) *Skill Mix in Primary Care: a Review of Research and Policy in the Past and Present, with Suggestions for the Future*, Occasional Paper 1. London: Centre for Development of Interprofessional Education (CAIPE).

Rink, E., Ross, F., Godfrey, E. and Roberts, G. (1996) The changing use of nursing skills in general practice, *British Journal of Community Health Nursing*, 1(6): 364–9.

Robertson, C. (1991) *Health Visiting in Practice*, 2nd edn. Edinburgh: Churchill Livingstone.

Robinson, B. (1993) Lyme cordial, *Health Services Journal*, 5 August: 20–2.

Robinson, J. (1992) Introduction: Beginning the study of nursing policy, in J. Robinson, A. Grey and R. Elkan (eds) *Policy Issues in Nursing*. Buckingham: Open University Press.

Robinson, J. and Strong, P. (1988) *New Model Management: Griffiths and the NHS*. Coventry: Nursing Policy Studies Centre, University of Warwick.

Rogers, A. and Elliott, H. (1997) *Primary Care: Understanding Health Need and Demand*. Oxford: Radcliffe Medical Press.

Roland, M. (1996) Defining core general practitioner services: a threat to the future of general practice, *British Medical Journal*, 313: 704.

Roland, M. and Wilkin, D. (1996) Rationale for moving towards a primary care led NHS, *What is the Future for a Primary Care Led NHS?* Manchester: NPCRDC.

Ross, F. (1996) Review of 'Prescribing the boundaries of nursing practice: professional regulation and nurse prescribing', *NT Research*, 1(6): 479.

Ross, F. and Elliot, M. (1995) *Innovations in Primary Health Care*. Edinburgh: Nursing Community and District Nursing Association.

Ross, F., Bower, P. and Sibbald, B. (1994) Practice nurses: characteristics, workload and training needs, *British Journal of General Practice*, 44: 15–18.

Ross, F., Rink, P., Godfrey, E. and Roberts, G. (1995) *Audit of Nursing Skill Mix in General Practice*. South West Thames Regional Health Authority Clinical Audit. St George's Hospital Medical School, Division of General Practice.

Royal College of General Practitioners (1992a) The founding story, in D. Pereira Gray (ed.) *The RCGP Forty Years On*. London: Atalink Ltd.

Royal College of General Practitioners (1992b) The institutional story, in D. Pereira Gray (ed.) The RCGP Forty Years On. London: Atalink Ltd.

Royal College of General Practitioners (1996) *The Nature of General Medical Practice*, Report from General Practice No. 27. London: Royal College of General Practitioners.

Royal College of Nursing (1997) *Nurse Practitioners: Your Questions Answered*. London: Royal College of Nursing.

Ruiz, B., Tabloski, P. and Frazier, S. (1995) The role of gerontological advanced practice nurses in geriatric care, *Journal of the American Geriatrics Society*, 43(9): 1061–4.

Ryan, A.A. (1996) Doctor–nurse relations: a review of the literature, *Social Sciences in Health*, 2: 93–106.

Salmon, M.E. (1999) Nursing research and public policy: enhancing effectiveness on a societal level, editorial, *Clinical Effectiveness in Nursing*, 2: 171–4.

Salter, B. and Snee, N. (1997) Power dressing, *Health Services Journal*, 13 (February): 30–1.

Salvage, J. (1992) The new nursing: empowering patients or empowering nurses? in J. Robinson, A. Grey, R. Elkan (eds) *Policy Issues in Nursing*. Buckingham: Open University Press.

Salvage, J. (1995) What's Happening to Nursing? *British Medical Journal*, 311: 274–5.

Scrivens, E. (1988) The management of clinicians in the National Health Service, *Social Policy and Administration*, 22(1): 22–34.

Secretary of State (1999) Letter to Christine Hancock, General Secretary, Royal College of Nursing. Department of Health.

Shepherd, E., Rafferty, A.M. and James, V. (1996) Prescribing the boundaries of nursing practice: professional regulation and nurse prescribing, *Nursing Times Research*, 1(6): 465–78.

Short, J.A. (1995) Dual perspective, *British Medical Journal*, 311: 303–4.

Sibbald, B. (1996) Skill mix and professional roles, *What is the Future for a Primary Care Led NHS?* Manchester: NPCRDC.

Silverman, D. (1994) *Interpreting Qualitative Data*. London: Sage.

Singh, S., Lloyd, M. and Webb, S. (1996) Focus should be put on barriers that hinder progress, letter, *British Medical Journal*, 312(20 January): 184.

Smith, R. (1996) A fund of changes, *Nursing Times*, 92(25): 31.

Smith-Regojo, P. (1995) Being with a patient who is dying, *Holistic Nursing Practice*, 9(3): 1–3.

Soothill, K. (1998) *Sociology Nursing and Health*, Foreword. Oxford: Butterworth–Heinemann.

Spitzer, W.O., Sackett, D.L., Sibley, J.C. *et al.* (1974) The Burlington randomised trial of the nurse practitioner, *New England Journal of Medicine*, 290: 251–6.

Spooner, A.A. (1995) A personal perspective: the psychological needs of spine injured patients, *Professional Nurse*, 10(6): 359–62.

Stacey, M. (1988) *The Sociology of Health and Healing*. London: Unwin Hyman.

Stacey, M. (1992) *Regulating British Medicine: The General Medical Council*. Chichester: Wiley.

Standing Medical Advisory Committee and Standing Nursing and Midwifery Advisory Committee (1981) *The Primary Health Care Team*. London: Department of Health and Social Security.

Starfield, B. (1992) *Primary Care. Concept, Evolution and Policy*. Oxford: Oxford University Press.

Starr, P. (1982) *The Sociological Transformation of American Medicine*. New York: Basic Books.

Stein, L. (1978) The doctor–nurse game, in R. Dingwall and M. McIntosh (eds) *Readings in the Sociology of Nursing*. Edinburgh: Churchill Livingstone.

Stern, T. (1996) GP benefits of nurse practitioners, letter, *General Practitioner*, September: 45.

Stilwell, B. (1991a) The rise of the practice nurse, *Nursing Times*, 87(24): 26–30.

Stilwell, B. (1991b) Defining a role for nurse practitioners in British general practice, in J. Wilson Barnett and S. Robinson (eds) *Directions in Nursing Research*. London: Scutari Press.

Stilwell, B. (1996a) *Pushing the Boundaries: Nurse Practitioner*, RCN Nursing Update, Learning Unit 065, pp. 1–27. Also published in *Nursing Standard*, 27(10).

Stilwell, B. (1996b) Patients' attitudes to the availability of a nurse practitioner in general practice, in A. Bowling and B. Stilwell (eds) *The Nurse in Family Practice*. London: Baillière Tindall.

St Leger, A., Schnieden, H., Warsworth-Bell, J.P. (eds) (1992) *Evaluating Health Services' Effectiveness*. Buckingham: Open University Press.

Strachan, R. (1997) Nursing teams benefit GPs, *General Practitioner*, January: 34.

Sullivan, S. and Pickering, N. (1997) *Patient and Carer Involvement in Clinical Decision-making: A Review of the Literature to August 1997*. Swansea: Clinical Effectiveness Initiative for Wales, Centre for Philosophy and Health Care, University of Wales.

Sweeney, K. and Gray, D. (1995) Patients who do not receive continuity of care from their general practitioner – are they a vulnerable group? *British Journal of General Practice*, 45: 133–5.

Sweet, S.J. and Norman, I.J. (1995) The nurse–doctor relationship: a selective literature review, *Journal of Advanced Nursing*, 22: 165–70.

Taylor, D. and Leese, B. (1997) Recruitment, retention and time commitment change of general practitioners in England and Wales 1990–1994: a retrospective study, *British Medical Journal*, 314: 1806–10.

Times Higher Education Supplement (1999) Universities receive booster shot, 16 July.

Titmuss, R.M. (1970) *The Gift Relationship: from Human Blood to Social Policy*. London: George Allen & Unwin.

Traynor, M. (1995) Job satisfaction and morale of nurses in NHS trusts, *Nursing Times*, 91(26): 42–5.

Turner, V. (1977) *The Ritual Process: Structure and Anti-structure*. New York: Cornell University Press.

UKCC (United Kingdom Central Council for Nursing, Midwifery and Health Visiting) (1992a) *Code of Professional Conduct*. London: UKCC.

UKCC (United Kingdom Central Council for Nursing, Midwifery and Health Visiting) (1992b) *The Scope of Professional Conduct*. London: UKCC.

UKCC (United Kingdom Central Council for Nursing, Midwifery and Health Visiting) (1992c) *Guidelines for Professional Practice*. London: UKCC.

Usherwood, R., Long, S. and Joesbury, H. (1997) Who works in primary health care teams in England and Wales? *Journal of Interprofessional Care*, 11: 225–7.

Venning, P., Durie, A., Roland, M., Roberts, C. and Leese, B. (2000) Randomised controlled trial comparing cost effectiveness of general practitioners and nurse practitioners in primary care, *British Medical Journal*, 320: 1048–53.

Vollmer, H. and Mills, D.L. (1966) *Professionalisation*. Englewood Cliffs, NJ: Prentice Hall.

Walby, S., Greenwell, J., Mackay, L. and Soothill, K. (1994) *Medicine and Nursing: Professions in a Changing Health Service*. London: Sage.

Ward-Miller, S. (1996) The psychiatric clinical specialist in the home care setting, *Nursing Clinics of North America*, 31(3): 519–25.

Ware, B. (1996) How acute and community nurses are sharing skills, *Nursing Times*, 92(48): 41–2.

Warner, M., Longley, M., Gould, E. and Picek, A. (1998) *Healthcare Futures 2010*. Commissioned by the UKCC Education Commission. Pontypridd: Welsh Institute for Health and Social Care, University of Glamorgan.

Watson, T. (1987) *Sociology, Work and Industry*. London: Routledge.

Welsh Office (1998a) *NHS Wales: Putting Patients First*. London: The Stationery Office Limited.

Welsh Office (1998b) *Better Health: Better Wales*. Cardiff: Public Health Division, Welsh Office.

Welsh Office (1998c) *Making a Difference: Research and Development for Better Health and Health Care*, Consultation Document. Cardiff: Wales Office of Research and Development.

Welsh Office (1998d) *NHS Wales: Putting Patients First – Involving the Public*, Consultation Paper. Cardiff: Welsh Office.

West, B. (1995) *Health Services Developments and the Scope of Professional Nursing*. London: Midwifery and Health Visiting Advisory Committee.

West, M. and Field, R. (1995) Teamwork in primary health care. 1: Perspectives from organisational psychology, *Journal of Interprofessional Care*, 9(2): 117–22.

West, M. and Slater, J. (1996) *Teamworking in Primary Care: A Review of its Effectiveness*. London: Health Education Authority.

West, M. and Wallace, M. (1991) Innovation in health care teams, *European Journal of Social Psychology*, 21: 303–15.

Whitehead, C. (1996) The specialist nurse in HIV/AIDS medicine, *Postgraduate Medical Journal*, 72(846): 211–13.

Wicks, D. (1998) *Nurses and Doctors at Work: Rethinking Professional Boundaries*. Buckingham: Open University Press.

Wiles, R. and Robinson, J. (1994) Teamwork in primary care: the views and experiences of nurses, midwives and health visitors, *Journal of Advanced Nursing*, 20: 324–30.

Wilkin, D. (1996) Principles of a primary care-led NHS, *Primary Care Management*. 6(7/8): 1.

Wilkinson, R. (1996) *Unhealthy Societies: The Afflictions of Inequality*. London: Routledge.

Williams, A. (2000) Review of D. Wicks Nurses and Doctors at Work: Rethinking Professional Boundaries, *Sociology of Health and Illness*, 22(2): 273–5.

Williams, A. and Sibbald, B. (1999) Changing roles and identities in primary health care: exploring a culture of uncertainty, *Journal of Advanced Nursing*, 29(3): 737–45.

Williams, A., Robins, T. and Sibbald, B. (1997) *Cultural Differences between Medicine and Nursing: Implications for Primary Care. A Summary Report*. Manchester: NPCRDC.

Williams, A., Cooke, H. and May, C. (1998) *Sociology, Nursing and Health*. Oxford: Butterworth–Heinemann.

Williams, S. and Calnan, M. (1996) The limits of medicalisation? Modern medicine and the lay populace in 'late' modernity, *Social Science and Medicine*, 42(12): 1609–20.

Williams, S.J., Calnan, M., Cant, S. and Coyle, J. (1993) All change in the NHS? Implications of the NHS reforms for primary care prevention, *Sociology of Health and Illness*, 15(1): 43–67.

Witz, A. (1992) *Professions and Patriarchy*. London: Routledge.

Wood, N., Farrow, D. and Elliott, B. (1994) A review of primary health care organisation, *Journal of Clinical Nursing*, 3(4): 243–50.

World Health Organization (1978) *Primary Health Care*, Report of the International Conference on Primary Health Care, Alma Ata, USSR, 6–12 September. Health For All Series No. 1. Geneva: WHO.

World Health Organization (1991) *Community Involvement in Health Development*, WHO Technical Report Series No. 809. Geneva: WHO.

Wright, S. (1995) The role of the nurse: extended or expanded? *Nursing Standard*, 9(33): 25–9.

Zarnow, R.A. (1977) The curriculum model for expanded roles, *Nursing Outlook*, 25(1): 43–4.

Index